For my
sister June — whose
memories may be
from mine

Patricia Atkin

AKA Patricia Crowther

SO LIFE GOES ON

Patricia Atkin

MINERVA PRESS
LONDON
MIAMI DELHI SYDNEY

SO LIFE GOES ON
Copyright © Patricia Atkin 2000

All Rights Reserved

No part of this book may be reproduced in any form
by photocopying or by any electronic or mechanical means,
including information storage or retrieval systems,
without permission in writing from both the copyright
owner and the publisher of this book.

ISBN 0 75411 168 7

First Published 2000 by
MINERVA PRESS
315–317 Regent Street
London W1R 7YB

Printed in Great Britain for Minerva Press

SO LIFE GOES ON

*This book is dedication to Len,
who encouraged me to follow my feelings and write
my autobiography and who introduced me to the writing
class. Also to all my friends and co-authors who put up
with my weekly verbiage.
Thanks to one and all.*

Preface

This is my autobiography. It is the story of my life seen through my eyes, described and related by me. My purpose is to relive my life, focussing on:

1. My family – its mores, its values, and the interfamily relationships as they appeared to me.
    George Johnston and Hilda Martin were united in Holy Matrimony at All Saints Church in Matlock, Derbyshire, and no man put them asunder.
    Thou shalt keep him in perfect peace, whose mind is stayed on thee. Let us be content.

    George   Hilda
            Patricia Anne   June Maureen

    Philosophy. Advance and gain independence through Education.
    Emphasis on woman's need to be independent and self-sufficient.
2. The environment in which I lived and grew up.
3. World events which affected my life and development, both mentally and physically.

As these weave and intermesh, I believe that I shall discover how I came to be me.

> You will never know how much enjoyment you have lost until you get to dictating your autobiography. Then you will realise with a pang that you might have been doing it all your life if you had only had the luck to think of it. And you will be astonished and charmed to see how like talk it is and how real it sounds and how well and compactly and sequentially it constructs itself and what a dewy and breezy and woodsy freshness it has and what a

darling and worshipful absence of the signs of starch and flatiron and labour and fuss and other artificialities.

Mark Twain

The Beginnings: 19 May 1925

Dinner was over and the young couple, now in the second year of marriage and excitedly expecting their first child, were settling down to enjoy a quiet evening with the wireless. Then it happened, severe and excruciating abdominal pains, just as they had told Hilda that this is how it would begin.

The midwife was summoned by the closest neighbour walking speedily to the midwife's house. There were no telephones in those times. In due course the midwife arrived on foot to prepare the couple's bedroom for this exciting, but scary event for which they had no experience – the arrival of their first child. The mother-to-be was settled in the old four-poster bed and the anxious father-to-be was constantly requested to leave his labouring wife to the ministrations of the midwife. The bedchamber now was no place for a man. A long and anxious night ensued, with labour proceeding very slowly.

By midday on 20 May 1925, both sets of grandparents-to-be had arrived. Now chaos ensued as everyone, in their need and willingness to help, created more and more tension and anxiety. By evening the midwife was expressing great concern at the lack of progress and finally decided that the family physician must be called. Now, the neighbours were well aware of the happenings in the Johnson household. Gaslights shone from every window, and there were constant comings and goings of friends and family. Then, finally, the physician's horse and buggy drew up outside the gate.

It was now midnight and another day had passed. There was still no baby. Finally, the physician decided that no further delay could be allowed, as signs of foetal distress were evident. Forceps were ready and the room was cleared of all but the labouring mother, the midwife and the physician. In the early hours of Thursday, 21 May 1925, the infant was delivered – a bouncing, healthy, nine pound baby girl – me. The agony was over and now the ecstasy began.

On 7 June 1925, at last, after two weeks of rest and care, both mother and infant were doing well. They were allowed to leave the protection and safety of the bedroom to begin their new life together. The first challenge was naming the child. Since I was the first grandchild to arrive in both families, this was indeed a challenge. After whom should I be named? Mother decided to honour me by naming me Ann after both my grandmothers. Emphasis was placed on Ann without an 'e' but in my adolescence and after reading *Anne of Green Gables* by Montgomery, I decided that I, too, should be called Anne with an 'e'. Mother was also determined to name me after her social idol, Princess Pat, a well known and adored society lady. Nobody complained and most praised her choice. My paternal grandparents were bitterly disappointed in my gender for they had so looked forward to the arrival of a boy, to ensure continuity of the family name. So Patricia became Patrick to the men in the family and Paddy the next best thing to my aunts. These nicknames were accepted by all and stayed with me for the rest of my life.

Finally the young couple were allowed to settle down to build a family life and soon settled into quiet domesticity.

Mother found housekeeping repetitive and dreary. Her emphasis on independence was ever present and she did everything possible to foster and support it in every way that she could through education, socialisation and travel.

My Home Town, Matlock

Matlock was a picturesque small town in the Pennine Hills, nestling along the banks of the Derwent River and surrounded by hills almost high enough to be considered mountains. Apart from the local limestone quarry and a mill, which manufactured knitting yarns, it had no heavy industry. Rather it was, and still is, a vacation haven and, in my youth, a well known spa. Three hotels were open all the year round. One called itself a hydro, a luxury hotel catering to people seeking relief from arthritis, a very common complaint and handicapping physical condition in England, by partaking of the local natural mineral waters utilised for bathing and drinking. Bordering the town were farmlands which extended to meet the hill country. With increasing elevation this turned into moorland. Nature was accessible to all who had sturdy legs and feet. At the time of my growing up, most country people did. Cars were a new-fangled idea, available to the very few and travelling for any distance was by bus and train.

Summer evenings in Derbyshire were very long. Darkness finally arrived about ten o'clock. We passed these long evenings by strolling after the evening meal, either through the meadows along the riverbanks or across the wilder terrain of the moors. Children of all ages accompanied their adults and were frequently seen riding pick-a-back or on a walking stick held at each end by the older members of the group. Their little legs could go no further!

As a treat families would occasionally stop for a bite at a pub or fish and chip shop. Walking induced an appetite and nothing tasted better than a bag of chips salted and vinegared to taste. The pubs, of course, were the men's domain. The women and children sat on outdoor benches. As I reached adolescence, some of the rural pubs opened a women's lounge where the wife and children could be served potato chips and soft drinks, whilst the head of the household socialised at the bar.

Everyone knew everybody else in Matlock. Most families had lived in their homes from generation to generation. Everyone knew both the good and bad about most family backgrounds. News travelled by word of mouth. In adversity, everyone rushed round to help. When my school hat was blown into the river one afternoon after school, my mother knew all about it long before I reached home to tell her. Most folk were born, raised, worked and died in Matlock. The cemetery had localised areas of family graves from generation to generation. Men in the family were the breadwinners. Women were homemakers and child-rearers and there was no deviation from these roles. Within the town there was great emphasis on togetherness. Class warfare was unknown. The doctor and the clergy were shown respect by one and all. Politicians were local men, with local ideas and tastes. They were one of us, and our friends.

Life was relatively carefree. People, on the whole, were satisfied with their lot in life and money and status made little difference. Everyone owned his own home and every family had its own garden producing vegetables and flowers, all for sharing with the neighbours.

A day spent in a neighbouring locality was always a special treat, but these were few and far between. Social life revolved around the church, the arts, the pub and for many – especially the men – sports, namely cricket in the summer and soccer in the winter. We had a small local symphony orchestra and an opera company. The annual performances of both were avidly awaited and overly attended. Picnics were a popular way to spend a Saturday or Sunday afternoon, alone with the family, with the extended family to celebrate a birthday or anniversary, and occasionally with a community group. Rain was the only enemy but this was so general that we all learned to live with it. Bugs and scorching sunshine were unknown.

Families on the whole stayed together and stood together. Everyone firmly believed in the adage 'United we stand – Divided we fall'. My family was somewhat aberrant. Father was raised in Yorkshire and all but he and one brother stayed in that county. Although he was accepted by the community, he was frequently teased about his alien origins. Mother was born and raised in Matlock. Her only sibling – a brother – had moved to London after World War One. My maternal grandfather and his second wife were very much a part of our family. We spent at least two evenings a week, dining and socialising together. After dinner, Mother would play the piano and we would sing the old country songs. Sis and I were encouraged to show off our talent. She sang and I played the piano. We were always given much encouragement, not always so well deserved, but nice to receive! So life went on in my early years.

We grew up in this peaceful and sheltered area, accepted and accepting. Through our daily interaction within the family and the school, the basic philosophy of life was conveyed to us. Despite the old adage that children should be seen and not heard, we were included in all family activities, even in some of the more appropriate adult discussions.

I can still hear Father ask, 'What do my girls think?'

Thus we learned the socially accepted mores for our successful maturing. Life was not simple. Everything was done by hand. Gadgetry did not exist. Food was bought, carried home, cooked and consumed on a daily basis. We read by gaslight and candlelight. Our washing machine consisted of a wooden tub with a dolly and a mangle. There was no clothes drier. Laundry was hung outside on the clothesline and there were frequent dashes from the house to take it inside whenever showers came out of the blue. Despite these idyllic conditions, surroundings and our placid life, the world was to change drastically and shake us out of our complacency.

The Families

H. W Madkin, my maternal grandfather, came to Matlock from Ashbourne to join Loverock and Son, drapers of Alfreton, a small prosperous mining community. After gaining experience in this field, he helped to open a subsidiary store in Matlock. As the years passed he became manager and later purchased the business from Mrs Loverock, following her husband's death. My maternal grandmother, Mary Ann Bradley, his wife, died in a diabetic coma early in my life. I never knew her apart from photographs and Mother's reminiscences. She, too was a woman before her time. She had been orphaned early in her life and had been put out to service in a local upper class family, the Padgets. As a result of this she was very aware of, and alert to, appropriately acceptable social behaviour, mode of dress, manners and deportment.

Mother would frequently quote her to us saying, whenever we felt devalued or misunderstood, 'Never mind their opinions. Just remember you are the Johnston girls.'

Both of Mother's parents believed in education. They had provided the best that was available for Mother and her brother; both attended a private school with fees. There were no scholarships in those days. Both went on to college. This was most unusual for small town families. Mother graduated from Leeds Training College as a certified teacher. This was very unusual in that day and age. She reminisced with much pleasure about her ability to leave home and find and hold down a job, and have her own bank account and her own pay cheque. She enjoyed the social life that this allowed her and the social contacts that followed. That was the beginning of Women's Liberation.

When the world was thrown into chaos by World War One, my grandparents persuaded her to return to Matlock, fearful lest she be injured or killed in the threatened air attacks promised for the big cities. Sheffield was particularly vulnerable as the centre of the English steel industry. She did return to Matlock, taught in one of the local schools and joined in the local social activities. She became an avid golf and tennis player, and it was through these interests that she met Father after the cessation of the war.

Father was the fourth in a family of seven. He was born and raised in Bradford, Yorkshire. His father, Albert, was a self-made man. He had the good fortune to manufacture flexible metallic tubing. Flexible metallic tubing was very much in demand during the war years and later in the post-war years and he had few competitors. He may have participated in its development as he had an inventive mind, but I never really knew if this was so. His logo was a globe with a cockerel on top and he was affectionately called 'Johnston, cock of the North'. Could this be the origin of my arrogance?

Grandfather developed a neurological disease and died when I was two years old. I thus only knew this grandparent through photos and family reminiscing. He believed little in education. He claimed that it made people soft and his philosophy was 'Where there's muck, there's money', alluding to the mining industry.

Father was seventeen when World War One broke out. He was still in school but he enlisted as soon as he was able in the RAF and became a pilot. He was quite proud of the medal that he was awarded, but he spoke little of his experiences apart from blaming his later suffering from fibrositis on an accident during one of his flights.

Norman, his oldest brother, took over the family business and became exempt from conscription. This was an ongoing bone of contention within the family as Norman later assumed ownership depriving all four brothers of any involvement in the family business. Following the cessation of hostilities and demobilisation, Father acquired a fluorspar mine in the hills outside Matlock and moved to live in the town. He joined the local golf and tennis clubs where he met Mother and, following a short courtship, they were married.

As Sis and I were growing up, we had a close relationship with my maternal grandfather and later after he had remarried with his second wife. Whenever we were on Main Street, we stopped by his store and were treated to a cup of cocoa or a candy bar which had been placed in a drawer just for us. No wonder that candy tasted so good. The store was a wonderful haven on a cold day as we awaited the bus to take us up the hill and home. We also spent Thursdays and Sundays together, dining at one or other house and enjoying music and our family singalongs. We both had great support and encouragement from G. P Madkin in all our endeavours, sports, school, music and art. I still remember how, after I became a doctor, he would always be at the train station to see me leave after one of those brief weekends at home.

He would kiss me and shake my hand leaving a pound note in my palm and quietly say, 'Be a good girl and have a little treat'.

Our relationship with our paternal grandparents was less intense because of the ninety miles between the houses. We spent short visits with Grandma and my parents, either at Cragg Cottage, the Johnston family home or at my parent's house, Kelvin Grove, lovingly abbreviated to Kelvin. As Sis and I became more self-sufficient and able to be independent, we spent our summer holidays with Granny, Auntie Win and Uncle Norman. The latter were father's older siblings, neither of whom had married. Both continued to live in the family house, until their demise.

I think I was eight years old when I was first allowed to spend time away from my parents. Sis was only four at that time and too young to be away from home. I remember some of the excitement and also the anxiety of that first separation. My uncle had a car and was to visit us, then take me back to Granny's with him. After the initial sorrow of saying goodbye, the journey was very exciting. We drove along over hill and dale at thirty miles an hour, which was the speed limit at that time. It took about four hours to cover the ninety miles between the houses. We stopped to get petrol pumped by an attendant, who expected a tip and, as the sun began to set, we arrived to find Granny's welcoming arms and Peter, the dog, yapping excitedly.

I slept with Auntie Win so that I wouldn't feel lonely. I still recall the big bed with its flannelette sheets, its plumped up pillows and the down comforter, all that even though it was August. None of it was superfluous. No other bed has ever felt so cosy and comfortable. The greatest treat of all was that I was allowed to retire with the adults. My uncle would be the last to retire and, before retiring to his room, he would stop to say goodnight and give a shadow display on the bedroom wall. Each day offered an array of excitements, but the routine remained constant throughout each visit and over the years. As I fitted in with this routine, I began to know that I belonged there, just as I belonged at home, and Cragg Cottage became my second home.

As Dad said, 'It's your home away from home.'

We arose at seven o'clock, toileted and dressed, and descended to find an English breakfast awaiting us. Nothing had ever tasted better than the fresh grapefruit followed by eggs and bacon, followed by toast and marmalade. Always there was a big pot of tea standing to keep warm on the fireside hob. After uncle left for his office, we cleared the table, washed and dried the dishes and then went outside to play, so long as the weather allowed. My playmate was the gardener's son, just a year older than I was, but very proficient in the physical accomplishments of boys of his age and generation. We ran, romped and wrestled together, walked through the woods with the dog and watched the trains go by. Sometimes, we would condescend to help his father with the gardening chores. My greatest pleasure, though, was to entice the lamb to be with us, by offering him an infant's bottle filled with milk. After a few days he learned to watch for us and then would gambol over to join us. My older female relatives considered this kind of play more appropriate for me – a young lady – and encouraged more of such feminine activities.

The afternoons were always spent with the adults. We would ride on the bus into Bradford, or on the train into Leeds and wander through my aunt's favourite stores. Every year, during one of these sorties, we were encouraged to select a dress for ourselves and our choices were usually approved. We couldn't wait for uncle to come home from the office to show off our new finery. Some days we visited relatives for afternoon tea. This necessitated dressing 'like little ladies'. Thus we learned the social graces of sitting quietly and speaking only when spoken to. This was so different from home, where we were encouraged to speak out.

Bedtime was always at ten o'clock. After the evening meal, usually high tea, as in England the tradition was to have dinner at noon, we made ourselves comfortable beside the fire, talking, reading, listening to the wireless, or playing parchesi. Our nightcap came at half past nine, regularly. Weekends were always fun. We usually took a trip on Saturday to a local event, or to a holiday site. We loved York, with its old walls and Minster. Walking on the walls gave me a deep feeling of awe, knowing that these stones had been there since Roman times. Everything had the look and feel of permanence, and this was very reassuring in that time of destruction and wartime violence. We were relieved when York was only minimally scarred by World War Two.

On those days when the sun shone and the weather forecast was good, we drove across the moors. There was nothing quite so satisfying. Here, we really felt close to nature. As far as the eye could see the wild terrain stretched to kiss the horizon. The country spread in all its glory of rolling hills, deep glens and valleys, windswept groves of pine trees, heather and little streams and rivulets gurgling over their rocky beds to the sea. No wonder the bards of earlier years, and more recent years, made their homes in this vicinity for some period of their lives.

We loved to picnic in one of the sheltered glens and we had fun identifying the specific one for that day. If it was too cold – and often it was even in August – we would be treated to lunch in one of the old inns. Here, everything was old. The old stone walls with their mellowness welcomed one, the old oak panelled walls gave a feeling of restfulness and the dining room with its white linen napkins invoked a feeling of elegance and luxury. When one's ordered food arrived, one knew what was meant by 'manna from Heaven'.

Sometimes, we went to the coast and, no matter which little town we selected, we always had a good time, walking along the cleansed smooth beach, tramping the rugged Brigg at Filey, or exploring the huge rocks and the little pools left by the tides with their little jellyfish and shellfish. All good things come to an end.

The days and weeks passed all too quickly. Soon it was time to return home. We were always sorry to say goodbye, but we were always happy to be back in our familiar surroundings and routines with Mother and Dad. We always agreed that it was great to go away, but that there was no place like home.

The Depression of 1929

I was almost four years old when the depression hit. I have no real memories of this time but, from hearsay, life became difficult and stressful for my family as it did for so many others. Father struggled against great odds to keep his business afloat and his employees at work. Despite his great optimism that 'It can't last for ever,' he could not beat the enemy. During this time, my sister was born and, although her entry into the world was less traumatic than mine, the extra stress due to the needs of another infant was hard on the family. Shortly after Sis's arrival, my maternal grandmother died in a diabetic coma and shortly afterwards, my paternal grandfather also died, the cause for which I do not know. He had been ailing and handicapped for several years, so his passing was not a surprise to the family but, for my parents, the recurrent losses of the main support figures in their lives was upsetting and hard to accept. To ease their grief and to find some solace for himself, Mother's father decided to move in with our family and I believe that he was a great source of strength to my parents, despite his own grief, during one of the darkest periods of their lives together. Just as Dad had predicted, the situation improved and he slowly recouped and successfully re-established his own business.

Whilst the adults in my life were under great stress, my own life was beginning to open up, for I entered school and this presented me with new vistas, new wonders and new ideas. Education was extremely important in my family. Whilst my paternal grandfather had minimised its value, believing as most Yorkshire men the axiom that 'Where there's muck there's money', my maternal grandfather believed that education offered not only security in life but also expanded one's ideas, beliefs and perceptions of the world. His mother, despite being widowed early in his life, had insisted that he be educated and he attended a one-room schoolhouse where his love of reading and music was stimulated and encouraged.

Thus for me, school and learning were an important and an exciting part of growing up. Both Sis and I were highly motivated to learn not only by our teachers but by our parents, as well. We were good students and so we were accepted and liked by our teachers. We knew them as people and they knew us and our family and they all respected Mother because of her education and, in fact, considered her as one of them. The only sour note was that my sister, who was four years younger than I was, resented having to follow me through school because of the expectation that she should be like me.

Our teachers set the curriculum and standards for learning but it was our parents who made it fun. We were encouraged to ask, 'How', 'What' and 'Why' and helped to find the answers from books and other resources and discuss our findings with them. Problem solving became a game in itself. Both Mother and Dad were avid readers and loved music. Some of my earliest happy memories are of being snuggled on one or other parent's lap and being read to by the fireside. Mother always read a story to us once we were in bed, and we often fell asleep before she had finished. As we got older, I took Mother's place and would read to Sis. Other early memories are of listening to classical music on the gramophone or to Mother playing the piano on cold and damp Sunday afternoons, beside a glowing coal fire and swaying or tapping in time with the music.

Both were avid country lovers. Flora and fauna were a constant topic of conversation and there was never a time that we did not watch the antics of the birds on the feeder during mealtimes. We always had pets, usually a cat and a dog, both considered family members and both given care by the children who were supervised by the grown-ups. We planted bulbs and house plants to cheer us through the long dark winter days and looked forward to the early blooming of snowdrops and crocuses and the arrival of Easter and its flowers, especially the traditional Easter lily which Father always brought home for Mother.

During my adolescence, my favourite uncle sent me six chicken eggs to be hatched. *How would we do this?* we wondered.

We decided to rig up a box as a little nest and to place it close to the coal fire, which we kept smouldering all night to maintain a constant warmth. Sure enough, one egg hatched and, in the morning, there was a fluffy little chick trying to stand. Shortly, he began to peep and, with our increasing attention, the peeps became louder. We all fell in love with this chick. What should we call him? we asked one another. We settled on Joey and he became an important member of the family. He selected for himself an old stuffed chair with a well worn hollow in its seat, in which he could curl up and sleep or rest. He always ate from the table after we had eaten, climbing up Mother's outstretched legs to her lap and pecking his titbits from the edge of the table.

Joey was a great watchcock. He spent his days roaming our walled-in garden and crowed raucously, whenever anyone entered through the gate. As he grew older, it was very hard to keep him in the house and it was reluctantly decided to ask the milkman to take him. This was as upsetting to Mother and Dad as it was to Sis and me. None of us had the courage to ask as to his fate.

During these years our daily lives followed a set routine, with school being the main focus for Sis and me. We had well defined rules, within and without the family, for our daily interactions with peers and adults and we all enjoyed the simple pleasures of life. Father was a great tease and his philosophy of life was built on many of the old adages: 'Never put off 'til tomorrow what can be done today', 'Have the courage of your own conviction', 'Live one day at a time', 'A place for everything and everything in its place'. He believed in taking the middle road and that moderation always triumphed.

Mother represented the down to earth, no nonsense aspect of life but, most of all, she was the comforter. She was always there, available whenever we needed her and it was her philosophic approach to life in general that carried our family through those crises that we had to cope with. Both my parents were optimists and now, as I look back over the years, I believe that this was their most precious gift to me. Mother's most frequent refrain was 'Laugh and the world laughs with you, weep and you weep alone'. We had all the essentials for our day-to-day needs but the emphasis in our day-to-day living was on sound relationships and personal interaction, rather than on material indulgences. One of our weekly treats was a bag of candy which Father brought home on Saturday and which stayed in his coat pocket until Sunday morning. As I grew older and wiser I discovered this, and would always check to confirm its presence when I made the early morning tea, which I took to my parents' room. Sis and I joined them and sipped along with them until our little tête-à-tête was interrupted by Dad leaving to start the fire and Mother subsequently joining him to fix our breakfasts – always bacon and eggs to ensure a good start to the day.

Because everyone was affected by world events and the scarcity of luxuries, emphasis was on survival as a group and helping each other rather than keeping up with the Jones's. So life went on with its challenges and its troubles, its joys and its happiness. Slowly the world returned to normal and we became more self-reliant and independent.

The Second World War, 1939

Ten years had passed and now I was an adolescent. Once again, the world was plunged into chaos and disorder as Hitler invaded country after European country in his efforts to dominate the world. England was an island fortress, protected from his army hordes by the English Channel. I remember the day that war was declared and how sobering this was for all of us. *What was going to happen and how would we cope?* we wondered. Father in his optimism said that the war would not last long, as our armed forces were superior to any in the world. How wrong he was! The conflict became intense and extended to include the Japanese and Americans, stretching the years out until the final armistice in 1945. Sobering as it was, the activities were also stirring and thrilling to a teenager. There was a great outpouring of patriotism, something we had not experienced before. The support, caring and concern for all enlisted men – not just for family members – at times seemed overwhelming. The world and our own environment changed overnight.

All lights were extinguished and blackout became a serious business, punishable if not adhered to. Local folk volunteered to be air raid protection wardens, whose job it was to check their patrol areas and alert any person whose windows showed even a glimmer of light. Streetlights were extinguished and only essential vehicles were allowed on the streets after dark. We treasured those nights, lit by the full moon. Matlock changed from a vacation haven to an army centre. The hydro was taken over by a high-level army department and the other hotels were converted into RAF hospitals. Social activities increased as the community attempted to fill the servicemen's lives with a little family comfort.

In Matlock, our day-to-day living was affected only minimally by the shortages of food, clothing and heat. In the urban areas, a black market soon developed, but this was minimal in rural areas where most folk were able to grow and store local produce. Our community resorted to the bartering of rationed goods. Nobody really went in need since everyone had something to exchange.

From time to time, our placidity was disturbed by the wails of the siren, denoting that enemy aircraft were nearby. This happened mostly at night. We would dress, stoke up the fire and play games to pass the time until the wail again notified us that 'All Was Clear'. It was my responsibility at these times to brew the inevitable pot of tea, always a ritual at times of stress, anxiety or worry. We would frequently hear the drone of enemy aircraft as they passed overhead and we occasionally heard bombs being dropped on the closest industrial cities. When Sheffield was under attack, we felt the vibrations of our old Victorian house as each bomb exploded in the city. One night, in the depth of winter we were shocked to hear an explosion close by. We all raced outside to see if there were any flames nearby and were greatly relieved that none were visible. The following day, we learned that a bomb had been dropped on farmland close by. It was reported that a farmer had been to his cowshed with a lighted lantern. There was no damage and no one had been hurt, but we all trekked off to view this thing called a crater.

The horror and gruesomeness of war was brought home to us sharply when we spent a few days in wartime London. The sirens wailed day and night and no matter where you were – even under the hairdresser's dryer – you were made to go to an air raid shelter. Of course, we all saw the funny side of the situation and joked about it, but this really covered up our fears and anxieties.

As the war wore on, we were subjected to the doodle bugs, guided missiles launched from the French coast. These could be seen and heard. The minute that the sound stopped, we knew that bombing was nigh and everyone, no matter where, prostrated themselves on the ground. These attacks were really nerve-racking and we northerners were lucky that the range was too short to interfere with our lives.

Throughout these years, we learned to become very self-sufficient, to appreciate whatever we had, materially and emotionally, but, most of all, the fact that home was always there. Because of our adolescence, my parents began to separate emotionally from us and to give us space and limits, clearly defining the boundaries between adults and children. We, as children, had our own well defined life now, our responsibility to go to school and do well, to get along together, to be loyal to and support each other and to help each other in times of need. Do our families today ever envision a time of need? Moderation became a way of life and we found this was both satisfying and rewarding. Another old adage that we lived by was 'Manners maketh the man – and woman', and we were expected to follow the social graces. 'Please' and 'Thank You' were important words in our vocabulary and we were expected to handle ourselves appropriately wherever we were. Respect for others was *sine qua non* and yelling and screaming at each other was 'verboten'.

As we matured, our family closeness continued but we were not overly demonstrative. We believed that actions spoke louder than words and we tended to meet each others' needs through the former. Physical contact – hugging and kissing – was confined to times of separation, goodbye and goodnight, and always carried the message that we would meet again, no matter what! This was very reassuring to a young person. Parental erotic feelings were not openly flouted within the family, although we adolescents sensed a 'something' between Mother and Dad in their subtle voice tones and facial expressions. We realised that there was something special between them that was special only for them. I remember thinking how great it would be to find someone with whom I could share such empathy.

We were encouraged to have our own private times when we

could do whatever we pleased. At night, we would repair to our own rooms to read or listen to music. Every Sunday afternoon, we each did our own thing for two or three hours with, or without, the others. Father loved his flower garden and often invited us to join him, but, if we declined, he was never offended. Mother loved to stretch out with her paper or book, and I liked to do the same. This permitted separation was good training for our own ego development and self-satisfaction. We learned that one can be alone but not lonely. One could find solace and peace within one's self, a sense of one's true being. Most of all, I learned that at times of stress or crisis one could quietly think the problem through, decide on the options for a solution and plan to act for the resolution. This training stood me in good stead in my adult years and helped me to weather several storms.

The family reunion occurred around the tea table. Mother always had a special treat, usually for one of us especially, but always enjoyed by all. Following this meal, our evenings were spent beside the fire with chatter and music. Mother played the piano and we sang the old favourite songs and arias from our favourite operas. I was encouraged to play my piano pieces and Sis would sing her most recent piece, in preparation for her presentation to her teacher the coming week. Everyone expressed their opinions of our efforts, not always totally positive, but I think this taught us that criticism offered within the framework of caring can be constructive and should be carefully considered. The empathy and emotionality of our Sundays completed our feelings of family togetherness and a sense of belonging, a valuable antidote to the alone experience. So the war years passed and life went on, but not before I was sixteen and needed to start to plan for my adult life.

Two events focussed my thinking. Whilst loss and death were ever present in war time England, I remember the horror of the illness with leukaemia of a schoolmate, Geoff Ruger, and his subsequent death. I still remember how debilitated and depressed he became and how important my daily waving was to him, as I passed his house on the way to school. This was always something to look forward to, as he lay dejected and lonely in his bed. His was the first funeral that I attended and I still recall the empty feelings each day as I passed his house and he was no longer there for me to wave to.

Not long after this loss, I remember witnessing an old man being struck by a car and watching the crowd gather and the ambulance men taking him to the hospital. We later learned of his death and, although I had not known him, I felt again a sense of emptiness. Were these two losses the origins of a rescue fantasy and did they programme me for a medical career? My subsequent interest in Lew Ayres in the Dr Kildare movie series finally clinched the decision and I was lucky to have the support of family and teachers to help me to follow my desires.

Higher Education

The meeting was over and the decision had been made. How important I felt that so many people, family and teachers, were interested in my future. It was almost overwhelming, as I reviewed in my mind all the compliments that had flown across the table. Most important of all, I knew now that I no longer fitted our headmaster's concept of the Matlockian intelligence, namely valementality – a word I heard over and over again but a word that I did not truly understand. As I look back now, I never did find that word in the dictionary and I still have not found it. I believe that it was his own invention. In discussing the origins with a friend, a classicist, I think it meant an inbred, insular way of thinking. This certainly would epitomise Matlockian thinking. Perhaps this concept helped him to cope with the frustrations that faced him in his work and in his daily living. For he was an intellectual, a Cambridge graduate and classicist, sunk down amongst the lesser intelligentsia that a small town like Matlock bred and hung on to.

How he arrived there I do not know, but he maintained his own standards within his family. His son and daughter, the latter a classmate of mine, both graduated from Cambridge. During the years of Mr Orme's rule, no other student from Ernest Bailey's, the name of my school named after one of its benefactors, had entered or considered entering medical school, so there was great support and encouragement from all the staff to help me to be successful. My acceptance would be an honour for the school.

The meeting consisted of Mr Orme, of course, and all my teachers as well as my parents. Father seldom attended school affairs, that was Mother's job and province, but his being there that day told me how much he wanted my wish to come true. As the meeting proceeded, and the group began to consider what assets I had to succeed in the entrance examination, it became clear that I needed more knowledge in physics, chemistry, botany and zoology. Mr Wagstaff, the head of the science department and one of my favourite teachers, pointed out that I had matriculated from the School Leaving Certificate and was therefore eligible to apply for any course in any university. Most people did not matriculate until they sat the Higher School Certificate two years later. This meant that I would be two years deficient in scientific knowledge and understanding and this would be very noticeable.

The euphoria now was over and I had to come face to face with reality. Nevertheless, he encouraged me to take the entrance examination at the University of Edinburgh, the medical school of which was the oldest in the United Kingdom and highly prestigious. To help me prepare for this examination, Mr Wagstaff arranged for me to take extra classes, which he himself planned and supervised. School started in September and I entered for the next examination in March. This was my challenge, exciting but very scary. Would I know enough after six months? Could I really do it? I thought of the speaker's speech at the last closing exercises, in which she referred to living life like the babbling brook, not drifting down and wallowing in the sluggish delta, but fighting it to the bitter end. Wasn't that my situation? I gave it all that I had. Study, study, study and more study. To take the examination I had to travel to Edinburgh from Matlock – a mere two hundred and fifty miles – but for England, and especially wartime England, this was a real challenge and the distance frightening for someone who found a visit to our closest town, Derby, some twenty miles away quite an ordeal, yet also an adventure.

My favourite aunt agreed to take me since she had fewer responsibilities than Mother. So it was arranged within the family that Uncle Norman would come for me in his car, take me to Granny's house and we would then take the train to Scotland from Leeds, a direct journey. The examinations were spread over three days and so we arranged to stay in an hotel, another first, new and exciting, but also a scary experience. War was still very much a part of our daily living. To go to Edinburgh despite the uncertainties – wow! What a thrill it was.

As I write, I recall little of this old city, just another old city with old buildings, old churches and parks. There was nothing new in all that! I do recall visiting the castle, yet another one, and having dinner at a restaurant, a real treat in wartime years, but my mind was too preoccupied with other matters and one specific goal to really take in the city's sights and sounds. Well, the arrangements were made and my aunt and I settled in the train with our overnight bags. What a symbol they became for me, for they implied the ability to move from one area of the country to another, with people to help us along. Now I began to understand what those holidaymakers enjoyed in Matlock. I think that first true journey must have given birth to my love of travelling and my yearning to see and visit places beyond the immediate environment.

It was a long and tiring trip and we were very happy to reach our hotel room in Edinburgh as the sun was setting. We ate in the dining room, having shared a picnic lunch on the train for there were no dining room facilities on the trains. After dinner, we were very soon in our beds and sound asleep, even though I was now beginning to worry about the examination and what this would demand of me. I sat for an examination each day and I knew that Mr Wagstaff was right. I needed more knowledge in all the subjects. I did my best to write good essays in those subjects of which I had a little knowledge, but I knew that they were not good enough, so I was not surprised to learn later that I had failed the examination. Of course, my pride was hurt and I consoled myself by saying that I was glad, because I did not want to go to Edinburgh; it was too far away from home. Nobody belittled me because of this failure, and Father suggested that the experience had been very good lesson which would stand me in good stead during my adult life. The school also decided that all was not lost and continued my extra classes. They recommended that I enter the first year of a BSc degree course and I entered the programme at Nottingham University, in preparation for entrance to a medical school the following year.

My acceptance by Nottingham University was one of the most important events in my life, for it ushered in the beginning of my adulthood. I left home – the first time for an extended separation – and lived in a women's dormitory, sharing a room with a peer, Maisie Sands, who was studying languages. We were quite different personalities and whilst sharing a room was a whole new experience for me, sharing with someone so disparate was a whole new challenge. Nevertheless, we became good friends and our friendship continued until she married and moved overseas during the post-war brain drain. I also learned a little about who I was. In my class were four other Pats and we identified ourselves specifically by using our first name followed by the initial of our surname. I thus became Pat J, later translated to Pea Jay, and so I acquired my third nickname. I had always been shy with boys. I was only seventeen but the male peers in our classes were all young adults, very sophisticated and women wise.

Socialisation was limited for all of us – again due to wartime conditions – but most of us allowed ourselves to attend the Saturday night hops. I became friendly with a classmate, Spencer Fields, whom I lost track of after moving to Birmingham. This was to be expected as I stayed focused on my goal, entrance to medical school. As the year progressed, it was necessary to apply to other universities with medical schools. I decided that I wanted to be within easy reach of home, and so I applied to the University of Sheffield and the University of Birmingham and I was accepted at both. Birmingham won, as the medical school had been rebuilt out of the city and close to the Licky Hills. This was for me. To awaken and see grass and trees, to hear the birds' dawn chorus and to see the seasons come and go was preferable to looking out on old buildings and city pavements with their endless hordes. So, in September 1943, and at the age of eighteen, I packed up my clothes and books and boarded the train to Brummagen, as the city was so fondly called by those who knew her. I entered another new and challenging chapter of my life, which was to last for six hectic years and terminate with a medical degree, the passport to a challenging, exciting and sometimes disappointing life and career.

The Birmingham Years, 1943 to 1949

Year One at Birmingham

The cab deposited me at University House, the hall of residence for women students. I was shown to a rather pleasant room in the main building with a high ceiling and large windows. It was already partly occupied by an attractive blonde girl. Her name, she said, was Jean – Jean Kennedy – and she had arrived just a few minutes before I did. She was to be my roommate for the first year. All first year students had to share a room. She would be my classmate for the next six years.

We greeted each other casually and formally and then we both set about settling in. This was not such a big job, as neither one of us had an excessive number of possessions. Besides our clothes, of which we had only the minimum – it was wartime England remember – and books of which we both had a few, mostly the same as recommended for the basic scientific subjects, I had brought an old travelling clock given to me my uncle. Jean had brought an attractive cut glass vase, a family heirloom, she said, which she kept filled with fresh flowers and greenery. No matter what the season, she always found some living plant with which to fill it. Later, she said that it was the fact that she could do this that gave her faith in life and its continuity.

My old travelling clock began a long and varied journey in Birmingham. When my uncle gave it to me, he had had my initials engraved on both the clock and its case – 'Just so it will always be with you' so he said – and he was right. My clock travelled wherever I did. I still have it, although it is only an ornament and a symbol. For whenever I look at it, it is like an old friend and reawakens many memories – happy and not so happy. It tells me that life is a continuity and that no matter what happens it must still go on.

After we had selected our beds and rearranged the room to our liking we were 'settled in'. When the bell sounded, we were glad to have each other's company and support, to face the horde of one hundred other young women arriving in the dining room for lunch. We realised the wisdom of the elders in giving new arrivals a roommate. We were introduced to the matron and the staff, who would be parent surrogates, and we had thoughtfully been placed at tables with others in the same faculty. We met three other girls, Lillian Jones, Jean Pearson-Wood and Margery Johnson who would be on our course and who would become our good friends. After lunch, we were free for the rest of the day and we arranged to meet the others at supper time. Jean and I had planned to indulge ourselves by walking around the area which was well wooded with green fields and narrow footpaths. There were no shops or stores to tempt us. The closest were a tuppenny ride on the tramway, which ran very close to the residence and made access to the village of Selly Oak fairly easy.

Slowly Jean and I began to discover each other. Our values and mores were very much alike and our goals and purposes, at least for the next six years, were identical. She was the daughter of a country physician, whose hope it was that she join him in the practice and carry on when he was no longer able. Her life was planned for her and she felt obligated to conform. For me, there were no plans beyond the coming six years, so I could dream to my heart's content. I wonder now if her inability to do this made her the rigid and lonely person that she finally became. We both loved the country and, whenever we could, we would take the tram to its terminus in the Licky Hills, roam through the fields and woods, throw ourselves down and gaze at the sky. If we could afford to, we indulged in a country tea at one of the few cafés or farmhouses offering such treats. If the weather permitted and we could eat outside, we felt even more satisfied. These sorties usually occurred on a Sunday afternoon for, the day after arriving, we were immediately plunged into a hectic schedule. From Monday to Friday, we had lectures from nine o'clock to noon and laboratory work from two o'clock to five o'clock. Our evenings were spent cramming or writing papers. Saturday mornings were chore times, laundry, hairdressing, etc. and on Saturday evenings we always attended the hops held in the Student Union, which was within walking distance of 'House'. This was very convenient, as there were no street lights to help us home after the event and we were always happy on those nights when the moon was full and bright and we could see where we were going, and also see who was being walked home by whom.

Attendance at the hops was crucial for a newly arrived student, for it offered the opportunity to meet with one's peers on a leisurely basis and also students from other faculties. Birmingham University was somewhat unique in that it had a faculty of brewing and it soon became apparent that the students from this faculty – all male – tended to like the women from the medical group. I never did know what the attraction was. We were, on the whole, a bunch of good-lookers, but there were many others from other faculties. We soon lost touch with these fellows for, after the first year, they dispersed to do their practicals and we got lost in the welter of activities associated with our courses. This made it difficult to arrange meetings since even weekends were soon incorporated into our academic lives and in those days nobody had a car.

Nevertheless, only a year or so ago, I met one of the brewers – younger than me of course – in Cambridge, where he was the brewmaster at Wild Goose Breweries and again, true to form, I lost touch with him. Whilst most of our days and nights were filled with academic activities, there were some opportunities to have fun. I met a fellow at one hop who was on the rugger team and I became an ardent fan, attending at home rugger matches and helping with the social activities that followed, but again, we lost touch because of our different and difficult to mesh schedules. One Saturday of every year stood out for both town and gown. This was 'The Day'. It was 'Rag Day'. The city went to great trouble and expense to prepare for student activities, ensuring that it was safe to wander the streets. Traffic was severely limited and only buses and trolleys were allowed. Nevertheless the citizens appeared in hordes and enjoyed the jostling and camaraderie of the students, all in fancy dress and all attempting to collect money for a deserving national charity.

These activities started at ten o'clock prompt and ended at four o'clock prompt. Prompt was prompt! A parade with floats and musicians was in place and ready to go promptly at noon, the route being cleared of any obstruction. During my first year, a group of women from our residence had opted to join a group of fellows from the male residence. They came to our residence and had tea and cookies. During this time, we introduced ourselves and sorted ourselves out at random. One very tall fellow dressed in army uniform but wearing an Arab headdress, invited me to be his partner. Off we went on shank's pony. In the course of our conversation I learnt that he was Bruce Pilley and that he lived in Bradford, not too far from Rawdon, my grandmother's home. So started a long and happy friendship. We met every Saturday night at the hop and when he left Birmingham University at the end of the year to rejoin his regiment, the Royal Engineers, we continued writing to each other and meeting whenever we could.

As we toured the Brummagen streets, we came upon a stray puppy. What should we do? After much debate, Bruce decided that he would take it with us. He carried it in his arms and we soon realised what an asset we had acquired, for we no longer needed to go to the people. They came to us, basically to pet the puppy, then deposit a coin in his collection box. Guess who collected the most money? What's more, our photo appeared in the evening paper. Bruce took the puppy back to his residence and was allowed to keep it in his room provided that he took it home with him at the end of term. Well, he did and the puppy became a family member for the rest of its life and no matter where we met, in subsequent years, the puppy was always with us. I wish I could remember his name!

So the year came to its close. We all took the examinations in June and we all passed. After the summer break, we all entered the hallowed halls of medical school. I decided to enjoy the summer vacation, since I had been warned by older medical students that this would be the last long holiday for the rest of my life. That warning proved all too true. So life went on.

Year Two at Birmingham

It was September 1944. I was now a medical student. Even though it had taken two years to make it, I was now there. Now, what was to follow? I returned to the residence after the summer break to find that I now had my own room in one of the building ells. On this corridor, my friends of last year had also been given their own rooms. We were all on the same course, had all the same classes and all the same schedules. What could be better?

I recall that short little corridor with great affection and my own room with even more affection. Now I had a few personal pictures and knickknacks – some had been Mother's when she was in college – which I could arrange just to my liking. I even had a teapot and this got much use over the next few years. It is still with me in my china closet. We heated our rooms by burning coal in the fireplace. We were allowed only one bucket of coal a week. How could we keep warm in war time England? we wondered. We soon found out, as the cold weather was upon us shortly.

My favourite aunt had given me a pair of warm slacks to help solve this problem, a pair that she had used on one of her cruise holidays. Despite Father's adamant refusal to allow me to wear them at home – ladies don't wear pants, or so he said – I changed into them after dinner and then wrapped myself in a heavy travelling rug. I wondered what Father would have said if he had known. Part of me felt a little guilty, part felt a little triumphant for I knew he really would prefer that I was warm. How to warm our hands was a problem. Only gloves really helped. We tried to share our fires, each lighting one on a given night and inviting the others to join in the warmth. Our friendships flourished under adversity and we began to share most things, good and bad. We all knew that that examination was not so far away and so we settled in the warmth and studied. There was no talking and no distractions. The next day we entered those hallowed walls.

There were sixty students in my year, twenty of whom were women. We were all from middle class homes, and we were all supported financially by our families. There were no scholarships in war time England. This changed in the post-war era. We entered the auditorium that first day rather soberly and subdued, for none of us really knew what was in store for us.

There were many new faces, for not all this group had taken the pre-medical science course at the University. Many from the local High School had been lucky to have had a comparable course in school. We were nearly all from the Midlands. This was the area that Birmingham University was meant to serve. We had two exceptions, Margerie Johnson from Trinidad and Tony Gale from Barbados. Birmingham University was helping to establish a medical school in the Caribbean. They selected students from the Caribbean area to study at the founding University in the hope that they would return to the infant University and help it along its way.

On this first day we all looked each other over and slowly began to socialise. We were all glad to have someone we knew alongside us too. Shortly after being seated in the auditorium, Professor Smout – known to us later and more affectionately as Charlie – the head of the department arrived. He was a rotund, balding man, very demanding, very precise, very cynical and very dramatic. He was always impeccably dressed and his long white coats always sparkled. I remember when he interviewed me for admission. He asked me why I wanted to be a physician. I replied with all the do-good clichés. I saw this was not impressing him at all and so I said that I wanted to be like Lew Ayres in the Dr Kildare movies. This did catch his attention and he asked me what I had seen that impressed me. I don't remember what I replied but he responded saying that he would visit the movies the next time a Dr Kildare film was showing. If he did, he must have enjoyed it as he did accept me.

Anyway, his lecture was our introduction to medicine and medical practices. He shared the history, the purpose and the ethics of the profession. In his final summation, he stressed what was needed to be done in the coming five years – basically we must keep our noses to the grindstone – to attain our goal. His final words, or threat, were that Birmingham Medical School would not accept or help anyone who appeared to be a square peg in a round hole, or a round peg in a square hole. After all, our University motto was 'Per ardua ad alter' wasn't it? True to his promise, or threat, four students from our year were sent down at the year end just because they were square pegs in round holes. Of course, we were all impressed and would frequently repeat this refrain to ensure that we wouldn't fit the bill.

The curriculum of this first year in medical school consisted of anatomy, physiology and biochemistry. Every morning we had lectures. There were two anatomy lessons, two physiology lessons and one biochemistry lesson each week. The afternoons, following the lectures, were spent in laboratory work appropriate to the lectures. This, for anatomy, was dissecting the human body. We were paired off – two pairs sharing the body – each pair being responsible for either the right or the left side. We had no preparation for this task. We all had mixed feelings and one's partner became one's bosom accomplice.

The first few sessions of wielding the scalpel were somewhat nerve-racking, but we overcame our aversion because of our group involvement and support. We were all in it together – so we could do all that was required to be done – good training for the years ahead! We sure used those after dinner sessions to express our feelings and to gain comfort from each other.

Gray's Anatomy became our Bible and Ernie Sims – a grey-haired obsequious little man – the guru of the dissecting room, became our confessor. Dr Brandt, an older man and a German refugee, was always available to us in our moments of need. Some gave pet names to their body, but I don't think that our group ever felt that friendly and intimate. We were lucky, as we had one male student in our group, Paul Hooper. He was a lively optimist, determined to be a surgeon. He was always obliging and willing to perform the hardest and most awkward task.

Evenings after dissection afternoons were always intense and we would cluster together in one room and quiz each other on the afternoon's work. 'Tell me the course of the aorta, or the vagus nerve. What are the attachments of the trapezius muscle?' we asked each other. These thoughts of the human skeleton preoccupied our minds. I remember going to the Symphony Orchestra concerts and trying to decide which muscles the conductor was using as he agilely flourished his baton. Physiology, of course, complimented anatomy. We learned the functions of our bodily organs and how they worked together. This was easier to memorise. Biochemistry was also difficult, despite our training in organic chemistry the previous year. The best part of the course was that this was our Friday subject, all day, lectures in the morning and laboratory work in the afternoon. For those who cared to bring lunch in a brown bag, there was a classical music lunch hour. I can't remember the professor's name, but I can see him now. He was always friendly to all of us. He never let us down. He always ended the last lecture with, 'Now, ladies and gentlemen, let us enjoy our lunch together with...' Here he would announce the name of the composer whose music he was to introduce us to that day. His assistant moved in and the music started. The programme had been planned with a specific point for discussion. It became an added learning adventure for me, as I began to learn why I liked or disliked certain music. Most of all I learned that music had to be part of my life.

Our social life was as full as our academic life, for we came to know each other as individuals, those who liked the same activities, those who were good company and those who liked us. We were a compatible group of sixty people, so it wasn't too difficult to find companionship for most activities. Although our Caribbean colleagues were somewhat different in their tastes, they were friendly and rapidly integrated into the 'club'. As the term wore on we were a pretty cohesive group, all with the same goals and purposes, to succeed and move on to the next course.

The Clinical Years

Pathology and bacteriology replaced biochemistry. At the end of the examination we all had passed. There were no more square pegs in round holes. We were now well versed in the structure and function of the healthy human body. Now we were to build on this knowledge base and discover how, when, where and why this magnificent machine went wrong. More importantly for us and for our patients, how we could put it right. As this idea began to sink into our minds, we began to have feelings of awe and self-doubts. Am I really going to be able to be a physician? we asked ourselves. Further pondering and discussion amongst ourselves raised many questions as to our abilities. Someone pointed out that was why we were here, to find out and learn.

Undaunted, we pressed on. Our professors, in their wisdom, had arranged for our ongoing clinical training to be both academic and practical. Our mornings now involved clinical instruction with a professor and or a registrar. We would muster in the appropriate ward at nine o'clock for ward rounds. We were joined by all the ward staff, sister, staff nurse and other nurses as well as the physicians responsible for the ward professor, registrar and houseman. We stopped at each patient's bedside, greeted the occupant and one student was elected to question him or her as to the current status of health. The history was related by the houseman to give a focus for discussion, a review of the clinical symptoms, diagnosis and treatment procedures, medications, laboratory tests, etc. being experienced at this time. We were enabled to see how and why the therapeutic response was occurring. This was wonderful training and practice for our later professional competence.

During those sessions, we grew to know some of the patients quite well and most looked forward to our visits, as they learned a little about their illness from the open discussion. Our evening sessions now became purely clinical. We would relate the clinical signs and symptoms of specific diseases and correlate them with the patients whom we had seen that day. Our afternoons were spent in systematic instruction, lectures in surgery, obstetrics, gynaecology, anaesthesiology, forensic and toxicology and pharmacology. In the three years from 1946 to 1949, we were taught the range of medical ills.

These included six months of surgical dressing, clinical and lectures. There were three months of casualty operative care, involving crises and emergencies, two weeks resident dressing in a surgical ward and two weeks resident medical clerking in a medical ward. During these experiences we lived in the hospital and were on twenty-four-hour call. This was an exciting but anxious time. It gave us a little taste of what was in store for us after we had graduated. That would focus on nine months of medical clerking, one month post-mortem clerking, one month of practical pharmacy, three months of obstetric clerking, three months of gynaecology clerking, three months of paediatrics, three months of ear, nose and throat treatment, ophthalmology and dermatology and one month of anaesthetics.

Courses in clinical instruction in tuberculosis, mental diseases, venereal and infectious diseases also took place. This was a formidable programme, made possible by the way that it was offered, through ward rounds, clinical classes and tutorials. At the end of the fourth year we passed the examination, the third MB in pathology and bacteriology. During this time, two of our peers contracted poliomyelitis, a disease that had been rare but which was gaining momentum. Sadly one, the girl Thelma Higginson, died. At the end of the fifth year, we passed the fourth MB in social medicine, forensic and toxicology, pharmacology and therapeutics. Our final examination covered medicine, surgery, obstetrics, gynaecology, paediatrics, infectious diseases, mental health and illness, venereal diseases and epidemiology. During this examination, which lasted five whole days, we were quizzed by oral and written examinations. Once again, there was much discussion and chatter amongst us as to how we had performed, what we had said, etc.

The results of the examination were to be posted on the Dean's notice board at a given time. Can you imagine the anxious times that we passed, chewing on our nails, recriminating ourselves and pacing the floor? Nobody slept, nobody ate, until finally – there it was – nearly all of us had passed. There were no square pegs in round holes. Utter chaos followed. There was back slapping, racing to get the use of what few phones were available and then it all settled down. Once again, awe took over. Now I'm a doctor. Now what? A job, of course, we thought. This sobering thought negated all the hysteria of the day before. Jobs were not available to all. Those students who had passed with the best results automatically received house surgeon or house physician jobs at Queen Elizabeth University Hospital. Alas, I was not one of the honoured few. Now the search was on. I was accepted at Dudley Road Hospital, the largest municipal hospital in the city of Birmingham, the fourth largest city in England. Life went on and my real medical career was to begin.

An Interlude Before the Plunge, a Month at Filey

I did not start until 1 July which was at least one month away. Now comes the packing up, vacating the room that had been a shelter and a haven for so long. There were so many feelings; relief that the goal has been achieved, fear of what was to come, and so many self-doubts. Did I do it and did I make it? I thought. There were so many goodbyes to be said.

I returned home and it was good to know that I would be there for a short while and not just another fleeting weekend. My old room was ready and waiting. It had its own ambience of welcome. Now, I could display some of my more adult belongings, truly making it all mine again. What we should do for fun and recreation became a family problem. Granny wanted me to visit Cragg Cottage and everyone agreed that I must. Mother had one of her good ideas, to spend a little time at Filey, the family summer home by the sea.

It was all arranged. I would go to Cragg Cottage for a week, then join Mother and Dad in Filey for two weeks, then spend the last days in Matlock preparing for my job. Filey is a small resort town on the east coast, sheltered in a pleasant bay on the North Sea. It is a very popular family holiday resort. August is usually its busiest time. That year we were there in June, long before the school and business holidays began. We avoided the hustle and bustle of holiday makers and we could enjoy the delights offered without long waits. Our apartment overlooked the North Sea and we could see international shipping on the horizon. It gave us a feeling of being connected to the world. Best of all, we could just walk one block into town and to the stores. Just across the road and one block down the hill was the beach. Filey's beach was perfect. The sand was washed by the tide twice a day and so it was very clean. It was delightful for walking and beachcombing was never dull. It always provided some treasure, an unusual artefact or shell.

Temperatures in this part of England are not conducive to sunbathing and swimming was usually a short in-and-out dip because of the low water temperatures. I can recall friends wading in the surf wearing winter coats. Filey offered other exciting pleasures. The Brigg, a large rocky promontory protecting one side of the bay, was a wonderful challenge for young and not so young. To navigate those huge rocks, especially when wet after high tides, was tricky and challenging. To poke around in the little pools and puddles, after high tide, was always exciting particularly when filled with water anemones that closed up immediately that they were touched.

Filey was a great place to curl up with a book, inside or outside, and after the intense life that I had just experienced I took every opportunity to catch up on the latest novels. Filey was a great centre to explore the coast, Whitby to the north and Scarborough and Bridlington to the south. Driving inland, we visited old houses which had stood for centuries, with their perfect gardens. Sometimes we'd get lost in the vast expanse of the moors. The peace and quiet of the isolation was a tonic that only the forced city dweller could appreciate. Overwhelming loneliness and fear were never present, for scattered throughout were old country inns with their public bars and dining rooms, where one could enjoy the local cuisine and meet the locals. Trying to interpret their local accent was no easy task. 'There's never now't but there's summat', was a well known saying. So the days and weeks passed and it was time to return to Matlock and prepare myself for the next chapter in my life – adulthood.

The Physician, 1949 to 1953

Adulthood

It was 1 July and I was to become one of the house surgeons at Dudley Road Hospital in Birmingham, the fourth largest city in England. Did I really make it? I asked myself again. It all seemed like a dream. No, it was not a dream. I was waiting for the train to take me from Matlock to Derby, where I had to change platforms to board the train to Birmingham. All went well and I finally arrived at the hospital. I was shown to the resident staff quarters and met the housekeeper. She showed me to my own room, a large, high-ceilinged, pleasantly furnished bed-sitting room. I was most impressed by the telephone beside the bed. It was almost as elegant as those in the Kildare movies! How my attitude would change in the not too distant future! Over the next few months the clanging bell would clang far too frequently, especially in the early hours. It became my bête noire!

I unpacked my suitcase and carefully, oh so carefully, hung up my long white coats and placed my stethoscope on a hook close by. I would never don that white coat without putting the stethoscope in its pocket. Without it, I would be lost. It was almost teatime and my neighbour entered my room. We had been classmates and we were glad to be starting our careers together. We went to the dining room for a cup of tea. We met our colleagues, a bevy of physicians, male and female, all new and in the same boat as we were, all starting a new chapter in our lives. We became a close group and got to know each other very well as the days and weeks rolled by.

After dinner, I retired to my room. Now I began to take stock. I was now on my own. I had a job and a pay cheque and a lot of responsibility. Did I really have enough knowledge and experience to succeed? I asked myself. Self-doubts assailed me, but I tried to reassure myself. Yes, it was true that I had been exposed to a wide range of medical experiences, even some very critical medical situations during my student clinical years. I recalled the time that we had been on ward rounds and one of the patients had collapsed and died immediately following her gold injection for rheumatoid arthritis, a very new treatment at that time. Also, the male patient who, just after returning from the operation room, began to bleed profusely. Thanks to excellent teamwork by nursing and medical staff, who dropped everything to come to his aid, he did recover. Always, I had been a bystander. Others had assumed the responsibility. Now that was to be mine.

There were three surgical teams in Dudley Road Hospital. I was to be house surgeon to Mr James Leather, later affectionately to be known as 'Jimmy' – the senior surgeon – and Mr Louis Aldridge, the junior surgeon. I was completely in awe of both, at first, but slowly came to know each as an individual with his own personality. Especially after a long day and sometimes an additional long night in the operation room, I was to be responsible for a male and a female surgical ward. Each had beds for thirty patients and there were very few days when we had an empty bed.

Twice a week, on Tuesday and Friday, I was responsible for all emergency admissions arriving at the Casualty Department. These cases covered the gamut of life-threatening situations, severe traumas, ruptured appendices, bleeding gastric ulcers, urinary retentions and so on. It was the hospital's policy that no emergency case be turned away. All too often this presented problems. What were we to do if all our beds were occupied? The medical director's response was to make beds, to put them up in the side wards, to use another team's beds until one became free on our ward, or to put beds in the corridor for less sick patients. We were constantly reminded that it was our duty to save lives and to make sick patients as comfortable as possible, until their recovery. Once the crisis was over, we could sort out the situation. Somehow, it always worked out. I believe that this was because of the camaraderie between all the surgical teams and at all levels.

Every house officer's life in this large municipal hospital was hectic and intense. Every moment of the day was accounted for. We were all on call for problems on our wards twenty-four hours each day and seven days a week. Our reward was one weekend away every sixth week. We were very much in contact with all our colleagues and came to know each other very well and under all kinds of situations, happy and not so happy. We turned to each other at times of concern for our patients and we covered for each other when we could.

My days began with a ward round with Sister, as close to half past seven as possible. We visited each patient, reviewed the chart of their progress and the recent laboratory work and made further plans appropriately, such as referral for occupational or physical therapy, etc. Then there was my routine scut work, obtaining blood samples, urine samples for laboratory tests, writing X-ray requests, etc. The nurses were not allowed to catheterise male patients but there was no similar taboo for female doctors. Most of the older male patients were embarrassed when I approached with the inevitable trolley, and there was great relief by all when we finally had a male nurse join our staff.

Once I was sure that all was under control on the wards, I went to whatever was pending for that particular day. Monday and Wednesday were operation room days. I assisted whichever surgeon was scheduled. This consisted of scrubbing up, and doing whatever was requested by the operator. This usually consisted of doing whatever was necessary to improve his vision, retracting, mopping oozing blood or clamping arteries. As I became experienced, I was occasionally allowed to suture the skin incisions, but never without supervision. No matter what my role in the operation room, it was my responsibility to follow each post-operative patient closely and I checked each one carefully, immediately they returned to the ward and before I turned in for the night.

On Tuesday and Friday, when I was on emergency call, the greatest problem was in communication. During those years, there was a telephone but no beepers or cell phones. Communication was by a system of lights. Each staff member had his or her own unique combination of red, blue, green or white. Mine was green and white flashing. When I saw this combination I sprinted to the nearest phone to find out where I was needed. Our lights in this hospital flashed rapidly and we believed that their message was 'Come on, hurry, hurry, hurry'. At the University Hospital, they flashed much more leisurely and seemed to say, 'Come if you like. There's no need to hurry'.

Thursday was outpatient clinic day. Here we saw old patients in follow-up services, evaluating their progress and ongoing needs and we also evaluated patients in need of surgical intervention, but not in crisis. These patients were placed on the waiting list, to be admitted when a bed was available. This clinic ended at noon. The afternoon was spent in catching up on records and laboratory work. Sometimes, I had no work to do and then I could indulge in a book, a game of tennis or a trip to town.

Despite the intensity of our lives, there still was time for fun and socialisation. Most of us were present at mealtimes and we were able to communicate with each other. Teatime was often fun, as we frequently enjoyed the company of the senior staff whom we got to know well, but never on a first name basis. There was a bridge group and a group of tennis players. Very occasionally, we would plan a movie or theatre trip but, too often, the group that did go was not the original group.

Nobody went home for the holidays. The hospital planned the festivities and we arranged our own little affairs. There were always little romances, mostly between the male staff and the nurses. My classmate, Sheila, did meet her Romeo. They were married at the end of their contract and developed a very busy general practice in one of the Birmingham suburbs.

The most stressful experience for me at this time was the loss of my first patient. How inadequate I felt! I had followed him post-operatively so very carefully, for we knew he was at risk. He was holding his own quite satisfactorily. I retired to bed long after midnight, knowing that he was in good hands with the nursing staff. Then the clanging of the telephone woke me. I knew what I was going to hear and I was right.

'Come, Dr C,' said the nurse. 'It's Mr Jones.'

I leapt out of bed and ran to the ward, but I was too late. I confirmed that he had left us, allowing the nurses to do their routine job.

Tomorrow would not be a happy day, for I must inform the relatives and meet with them as early as we could arrange. How would I tell his family the sad news? Nobody had talked of, or prepared me, for this aspect of a physician's life. I lay in bed planning the scenario. As soon as I could, I went to the dining room in the hope of finding one of my colleagues there. Just as I had hoped, Jim, one of the most experienced housemen, was there. He knew just by my demeanour what had happened and invited me to sit next to him and 'spill the beans'. He knew just how to talk to me and, as a result, I was able to be supportive to the Jones family. Of course, I didn't ease their grief, but at least I didn't increase their stress and misery. As I think back to that sad experience I realise how wise and helpful Jim had been. He helped me to face up to and work through my own anguish, rather than lecturing me. So I learned that good teaching comes only from the ability to profit from experience, whether it be one's own experience or that of someone whom one can trust.

As I relived this time, I realised what a wonderful preparation for adulthood this surgical job offered me. I learned to organise my life, to develop priorities, to recognise and follow through on my responsibilities and to know when I needed to turn to my seniors for help. Mr Aldridge turned out to be the best friend that I ever had. Whenever I called him he came, no matter what the time or place, and he never belittled me. Rather, he reassured me that I had done the right thing. No wonder I was sad to say goodbye to the surgical group, but how lucky I was that my growth was to continue as a house surgeon to the obstetric and gynaecology unit in the same hospital and with my new-found friends and colleagues.

The Second Job

The 1 April 1950 was transfer day. I would now be one of the house surgeons to the obstetric and gynaecology unit. There was no need to pack up and move. Now, instead of running down the long corridor in the old building, I would need to run across the grass to the brand new building – just recently opened – housing both departments. Everything, everywhere, glittered and shone and the floor plan was very convenient. It was easy to move from one section to another, from the outpatients to the wards and to the delivery room for they adjoined each other. Nobody could appreciate how helpful this was unless they had experienced the need to be present in two places at the same time.

Mr Wentworth Taylor was the senior obstetrician and gynaecologist, a kindly, introverted man dedicated to excellence. He was our boss and we knew it. There was no nickname for Mr Wentworth Taylor. We all trod rather solemnly when he was there but, of course, we realised that his was not an easy job. Now, we were both responsible for not one, but two patients, the mother and her child. Whilst Mother Nature took care of birth very effectively on most occasions, there were times when she played some pretty nasty tricks. No wonder he was a solemn man. How sorry I am that I never got to really know the man behind the mask.

Our registrar was Morag, a very pretty, petite, vivacious woman with a broad Scottish accent. She was just a little older than we house surgeons, but she had already made her commitment for life. Patrick – Pat – McGibbon was the other house surgeon, an intense Scot, who was teetering on the brink of committing himself to a lifetime of obstetric and gynaecology. Such commitment could not be taken lightly. For in this specialty, one was really committing one's life totally to the job, on call twenty-four hours a day, seven days a week and fifty-two weeks a year. Babies arrive when they arrive and sometimes under very life-threatening conditions. As physicians, we were committed to being available to our patients, no matter what, during this dramatic event in their lives. We had a wonderful nursing staff directed by Sister Cotton. All were trained midwives and all were well versed in the limits of their skills. If they called you, you had better go. Something serious was cooking.

On arriving at the delivery room, the labouring mother was made as comfortable as possible by the midwife, usually known to the patient through the mother's prenatal visits. Routine practices and procedures were begun. Every four hours, blood pressure and pulse rates were charted, and the frequency of labour pains recorded as well as levels of comfort and tolerance. As the frequency of the pains increased, the physician was called to determine the progress of the labour. This was estimated by measuring the dilatation of the cervix and the descent of the infant's head into the pelvis. At the appropriate time, the midwife would encourage the mother to strain in sync with her labour pains. Progress was monitored by auscultating the foetal heart sounds and following the progress of the descending foetal head. Usually the birth was completed without any contingencies, for most of the women who came to Dudley Road Hospital had been regular attendants at the prenatal clinic and so we were all aware of those patients at risk from the clinic report. Even so, the physician was called when delivery was imminent; so that he was on hand to check the new-born infant and render any needed services.

There was always a feeling of elation and satisfaction when one could present a normal, full term, healthy infant to its mother and witness her reaction to this new addition to her life. It wasn't until years later when I had my own child, that I could begin to appreciate the relief and happiness that surged in the mother as her long nine month gestation was resolved successfully. No male could ever understand this aspect of birth.

At the time of my obstetric and gynaecology house job, fathers were not encouraged to be part of the delivery, although most of them brought their wives to the hospital and hung around, pacing, fussing, smoking and keeping others in the same boat company as best they could, until the event was over. It was always satisfying and reassuring to see the little trio united for the first time. This made working in this specialty such a satisfying experience, but then, of course, there was the other side. Occasionally a pregnant woman, unknown to us, would arrive in a life-threatening state. This was usually due to profuse bleeding, always a worrying situation. Routine practices and procedures were followed and the patient was admitted to the operating room. Morag was called. Just her arrival would bring calm and order and relieve the tension that always accompanied these cases, but we had already got the situation under control. An intravenous injection had been started and the mother calmed with a dose of morphine. Now Morag would do her own assessment of the situation and prepare for whatever had to follow. This usually meant a Caesarean section to deliver the infant and do whatever was needed to stem the bleeding. In most cases, the mother survived. Often, the infant would be at risk because of prematurity. At this time we had few aids to sustain premature babies. At Dudley Road Hospital, we were fortunate to have a special ward for these little infants with a paediatrician specialised in their care, and a staff of nurses with special training and experience. We house surgeons were happy to be relieved of the infant's care and to be able to devote our skills to fostering the mother's recovery. Much later in my career, I worked with Dr Victoria Cross, Vicky to her friends and colleagues, and one of the first pioneers in premature infant care.

At the time, I was doing this house job, it was the practice to coddle the mothers. They were kept in the unit for seven to ten days post-natally, partly to reduce the risk of infection since there were no antibiotics then, but also because we firmly believed that rest was a very necessary prerequisite for healing and return to health. During this time, the new mother was taught how to care for her infant, feeding hygiene, stimulation, etc. and to have a feeling of confidence to carry on at home. For during her time in the hospital, mother and child were given the opportunity to focus on each other with no extra demands intruding on their time together. I now believe that this fostered the mother–infant bonding, so necessary for the child's ongoing development. Today, mothers are sent home as soon as possible after delivery and they are expected to cope, not only with the new arrival but with all the other aspects of their living, before they have had a chance to catch their breath and reorient themselves to another responsibility for which many are ill-equipped. So much for my obstetric experience.

Gynaecology was much less stimulating. We helped Mr Wentworth Taylor in the operation room, having prepared the patient for this ordeal. Clients were admitted from outpatient clinic waiting lists. Pre-operative evaluations were done and surgery followed. Mr Taylor operated on two days each week and it was our responsibility, as it had been in surgery, to make the post-operative patients as comfortable as possible. These patients were older women, frequently being repaired for the damage done to their bodies by childbirth. Occasionally we would admit a young woman who was miscarrying, or who was bleeding because of uterine pathology. These patients frequently reappeared in the obstetric clinic shortly after expecting another child, and so life went on and thus 1950 passed for me. I learned to understand the human body and the humans inside those bodies, the situations that they encountered in their daily living and the ongoing need expressed by so many for continuity. I did not understand all of this but much, much later in my own life, it began to make sense.

The House Physicianship

I was now house physician to Dr Kenneth May – senior consultant – and Dr Richard Gillespie – junior consultant. This was my third job. How time had passed. I was almost beginning to be a well experienced doctor. I can recall little of this job and its challenges and I have no photographs to jog my memory. Dr May was every bit the physician. Elegant, highly polished, immaculately dressed but quite aloof. Dr Gillespie – Dickie to his friends – was a dour Yorkshireman with whom I could relate well. I understood his background, his gruff exterior and the reason for it. After all, was I not half Yorkshire?

I recall, when we met, that he said something to the effect that he hoped I didn't mind hard work. I responded with a real Yorkshire accent and dialect. After that, we were friends. It was as the result of this positive relationship that one of the most important events of my life occurred, which was to have great influence on my future.

As the job was coming to its end, Dickie raised the inevitable question that I had been avoiding: 'What are you planning to do now?'

I had no answer for I had no goal or purpose. Anyway what did it matter? For there were few jobs available for physicians, other than those returning from the war.

As we sipped our coffee, he dropped the bombshell. Yes he knew the job situation. Yes, he knew the priority for my group to get a job was low.

So – and here it came – 'Why don't you plan to go over to USA for a year? You are footloose and fancy-free and what can you lose – and more important – what can you gain? One year in a progressive country!'

My first response was 'You must be daft,' a Yorkshire expression used whenever what was suggested was totally inappropriate. What would my family say and how would they feel?

Unruffled he said, 'It's only a commitment for one year.'

Well, he had started me thinking about what to do and he had given me a focus. He even told me how to go about doing it.

'Look in *The Lancet*,' he said. 'There are several places looking for well trained English doctors.'

I did look in *The Lancet*. There it was.

Well trained English doctor needed at Vassar Brother's Hospital in Poughkeepsie, New York.

Out came the atlas. It was not a bad location. Poughkeepsie was on the Hudson River, about one hundred and ten miles from New York City. It was a small college town. Vassar College was located on the outskirts, founded by the Vassar Brothers with money made from brewing. The town was in Duchess County, for the most part a semi-rural area. I called home and, as expected, my parents were shocked, stunned and quite upset.

Mother's immediate response was, 'Well, I never, going so far from home and to a foreign land.'

Dad was rather quiet and sad. 'Well, let's think about it and we can talk when you are next home,' he said.

The weekend that I was home, we were gathered for family dinner. Conversation was general.

Then out of the blue, Father said, 'Pat, I've been thinking about your going to America.'

Everyone stopped whatever they were doing or saying and fixed their gaze on him.

'It will be a real adventure for you, both personal and professional. You have no commitments here. So what can you lose? It's an opportunity that you should not pass up. The time will fly and you will be home before we know it!' What a commotion there was at the table but, when order was restored, everyone agreed with Dad!

Investigation with the Immigration Authorities proved that I could enter the USA for one year only, on a special visa, Then I had to return to England. So there was some control in the situation and I couldn't go gallivanting, even if I was so inclined. If

I did want to return to the USA to work, I had to commit myself for five years and declare a willingness to become a citizen. It all seemed just right for me to have one year away from home Everyone agreed. The letter was written and mailed to Vassar Brother's Hospital in Poughkeepsie, New York, USA. Meanwhile, we all followed our regular routines, for nothing could change or happen unless they accepted me. So I awaited the mail each day, with bated breath.

The American Adventure, 1953 to 1954

The Turning Point

Finally, the long awaited letter from America arrived. How many weeks had it been? How many days had we had high hopes, only to be dashed by the postman's visit? How often had we said that 'No news is good news'? Was it? Now all would be revealed. I fumbled to open the envelope – certainly well and truly sealed – with my stomach churning and my heart aflutter. It said:

> *Dear Dr Johnston,*
> *Yes, we would like to have you on our staff for one year, starting on*
> *1 July, or as close to it as possible.*

Yes, no news was good news. I was stunned. The opportunity had arrived and I had to make the most of it. Still, I was ambivalent. To leave home and all that I knew and understood, all the people that I loved and cared for, and who cared for me. Should I go? No matter how hard I tried, I could find no reason to say, 'No!' That night I called home, just to be sure that we all agreed. We did. Now followed all kinds of frenzy.

I contacted the Immigration Authorities who agreed to the one year visa. 'How long would it take to receive it?' I asked. The bureaucrats could give me no answer. Then I had better wait until it was in my hands before trying to book a passage, I thought.

Transatlantic travel in the post-war years was very meagre. Air travel was very limited and only for the very rich. Average folk in England depended on the ocean-going liners of the Cunard fleet. This consisted of several small to medium-sized vessels ploughing the Atlantic Ocean between Southampton and New York, the journey taking five to seven days. When the visa arrived, I contacted a travel agent to arrange the passage. I would sail on the *Mauretania*, a 36,000 ton ship due to arrive in New York on 3 July.

Little did I know what that would add to the adventure.

The acceptance letter was dispatched to Vassar Brother's Hospital and I was ready to go. I had to pack up, get my belongings home to Kelvin Grove and repack for America. We sorted through the clothes. All were pretty shabby.

'Just take the necessities,' said Mother, 'and build your wardrobe when you get there.'

I didn't tell her that I was only allowed to leave England with thirty dollars in my pocket. I would accumulate things slowly, as I earned. There was so much excitement these days but, oh, so much sorrow!

Everyone put on as good a face as possible but nobody fooled anybody. I was taken to Southampton by my parents, my sister and my uncle and aunt. Reservations had been made at the Polygon Hotel and we were driven in my uncle's car from Matlock to Southampton. Could we make it in one day? we thought. We left early, about six o'clock. We would be there in time for dinner if all went well. There were no big highways in those days, no ring roads and the speed limit was thirty-five miles per hour.

We did it. Again, everyone tried to make light of the pending separation. What an adventure this was to be! Dinner came and went, then bedtime. Sleep came reluctantly. Tomorrow came and it dawned a beautiful day. This was the day that we had all anticipated and dreaded. We arrived at the assigned dock at the assigned time. My luggage was stowed and we sat together watching the commotion of preparing a transatlantic liner for its journey. It was a new experience for all of us. My aunt had travelled throughout Europe and had on occasion sailed from Southampton, but she had never experienced anything quite like this.

Then it came, 'All aboard, all aboard.' My heart flipped over. Hesitantly, I rose and reluctantly kissed and was kissed by everyone. Mother hugged me closely, wished me 'Bon Voyage' and a happy year. 'Don't forget to write,' was her usual plea whenever we were separating. I promised to send weekly letters, just as I had always done since leaving home. Everyone promised to write to me. I climbed the gangway and rushed to the deckside to wave for as long as I could.

Now the parting was over and I was all alone. I decided to go to my cabin. The luggage was neatly waiting to be unpacked and my cabin mate – of whom I have no memory – was settling in. I remember little of the voyage. We arrived in New York in the late afternoon of 3 July. What chaos and confusion! It was an utter madhouse, as people were all intent on getting a place for the holiday tomorrow. We coped with all the formalities of arriving in a foreign land. Now came the problems! How could I get to the railroad station? With a little help from a policeman I got into a taxi, and what a ride I had. There was traffic like I had never seen before. Frenzied drivers were trying to beat the traffic lights. At last, Grand Central Station came in sight and more madness occurred. I had no idea of the value of the strange money. I paid the cabby his fare, and then I gave him a quarter for his tip. A flood of verbiage followed and he flung the quarter into the gutter and drove off. Oh well! I guess you can't win them all. I recovered the coin. Now to find the train to Poughkeepsie, another taste of chaos and confusion, but I did it.

The ride along the Hudson River was relaxing and pleasant. It was just a taste of what was to come later in the year. Eventually, I was standing on the platform in Poughkeepsie, then in the hospital lobby. I reached my own room and eventually went to bed and fell asleep. Tomorrow was another day and it would dawn soon enough, I thought. So, life went on.

Surprise, Surprise

Tomorrow has finally arrived. A soft early morning glow filled the room as the sun started to peak out of the east. I felt no jet lag but then, this phenomenon was not known at that time. I would get to know it very well as the years went by. I made myself ready and went for breakfast with some trepidation, for now I was to meet my colleagues and messmates. The dining room was small and cosy with several tables laid for four, ready and waiting.

I saw one woman doctor sitting alone at one of the tables and I joined her. She was tall, very blonde and very friendly. She was impeccably dressed in the required white blouse, white skirt and white coat. She had a very heavy accent – German, I think. Her name was Marga – Marga Lottermoser. She was welcoming and made me feel at ease. The waitress arrived with the menu and quickly brought my order. As we joked about our preferences for tea and coffee, two older male physicians arrived and joined us. They, too, were friendly and welcoming. Both had heavy accents, Latvian, they said. Both had noticeable difficulty in understanding the conversation. I was beginning to understand the emphasis in the advertisement for English doctors.

Slowly the room filled up. Everyone greeted me. Then I felt hands on my shoulders.

A voice that I remember well said, 'Welcome to your new land,' and a kiss was planted on my cheek. I couldn't believe my eyes. There stood Peter Goode, one of my classmates. He joined our group and there was much excitement and chatter. He too had been encouraged by Dickie Gillespie to look in *The Lancet*, and had been at Vassar Brother's Hospital for the past six months. The hospital administrator, I learned, had alerted Peter to my application and had accepted me on his – Peter's – say so, or so he said. Anyway, what a wonderful surprise it was! Peter knew his way around the hospital, the town and New York City, the city of his dreams and the place that he visited whenever he could. He had also developed as friends a group of British people who were working at other hospitals in the area. I was quickly integrated into both the professional and social life of the hospital and I had little time to feel so far away from home.

My professional responsibilities were much the same as in England. Because I had no language problems and because of my extensive experience with both medical and surgical conditions, I was made emergency room doctor. This was ideal and added to my professional growth. Here, I had to ride the ambulance whenever it was called. I was at the scene of accidents on highways, in homes, hotels, stores, in fact wherever they occurred. It was my responsibility to get the patients from the scene back to the emergency room, then make decisions for treatment. Senior staff members were always available to me but I seldom needed their help. Slowly, they came to respect my judgement and I soon realised that Birmingham had trained me very well.

I gained entry into all kinds of places that I would never have had the opportunity to see, taverns, homes of both very rich and very poor, work places, even the local bordello, when one client suffered a heart attack. I even got into the local jail. Mother had always said that one half of the world didn't know how the other half lived and I was beginning to see how right she was. One big advantage was that I had only one night duty a week!

On one of those nights, in the depth of winter, we were called to pick up a man crawling in the gutter and who could not be restrained. Off we went. After much searching, we found him in a gutter which had become a stream. The ambulance driver, assisted by a local policeman, managed to get him into the ambulance. Then it was my job to look after him, until we arrived at the hospital. He fought and struggled, as we attempted to restrain him. Then he gave me a hearty shove with his foot and sent me flying out of the ambulance to land in a big puddle just waiting for me. How was I going to manage this man on my own? Both men knew that I could not do it without sedating him, but sedation would only delay diagnosis and treatment. Without more ado, the policeman called the station and was freed to ride with me in the ambulance.

When we reached Vassar Brother's Hospital and were able to evaluate him, the patient appeared to be psychotic and in need of hospitalisation at the State Hospital. Whilst arrangements were being made for his admission, I lightly sedated him for I had to ride with him again and this time with no assistance. Our trip out was uneventful. We were kept waiting for a whole hour before the admitting doctor arrived and the sedative was beginning to wear off, sufficient for our diagnosis to be confirmed. He was admitted to their emergency ward, where he had every facility at hand.

In talking to this physician, I discovered another British person. Recently arrived from England, he and his wife joined our group. We met often and got to know each other. Our friendship continued for many years. Joe and his wife moved to New Bedford, Massachusetts, where he developed his own practice and I spent many happy weekends with them in their new home. We lost touch with each other after I married, when another whole new world opened up for me, many years later. Thus started a new year, in a new land and culture. It promised to be another good experience. So life went on.

A Year in Duchess County, New York State, June 1952 to 1953

The following day was 4 July. I had been there now for twenty-four hours. It was a holiday and I had not been assigned to work. I had unpacked and cased the hospital and locality. Now, I had some sense of direction. It was twilight and night was settling in and I was sitting on the terrace overlooking the Hudson River. What was that? There came a sudden flash and then another and another, then a whole panorama of flashing lights through the trees. What a breathtaking spectacle, that repeated and repeated. What was I seeing? I had never seen anything like this before.

A woman walking towards me stopped and joined me to watch the splendour. We exchanged comments and I learnt that I was witnessing fireflies in their summer activities, something that I had never seen, or known about. Later, I learned that my companion was on her way to see the holiday firework display. Well, I had had my own celebration with the fireflies. I silently wished Dad, a happy birthday for this was his natal day. What a shame that he could not be with me to witness nature's spectacle. He would have enjoyed it so.

The following day arrived and I was integrated into the hospital staff. The usual medical and surgical problems were challenging, as always, but were treated much as in English hospitals. During this year, I met many people and made many acquaintances, but three special women became my lifelong friends. Marga, the other female intern and I were naturally drawn together. We ate together whenever we could, swapped our clinical concerns and practices, and socialised very occasionally. We liked and respected each other despite our different nationalities and got along very well, but there was always an aloofness between us. Was it the language? We really didn't have time to think about this until Christmas Eve when Marga invited me to celebrate her Christmas with her. As we were enjoying the wine and goodies, Marga quietly said how terrible the R.AF attacks on Essen and other German cities had been. There was no threat or accusation in her voice, just a statement of fact. I replied in kind. I described how terrible the Luftwaffe's attacks had been on Coventry and Sheffield, to name only two cities and how, during the attack on the latter city, I had been sick in bed with measles and our old house ninety miles away had rocked as each bomb exploded. There was no challenge of right or wrong from either of us.

We both realised that we had shared similar experiences of fear and destruction as victims of powerful governments. This was the beginning of a lifelong friendship. We have kept in touch over the past forty years and have met whenever we could. At those times it was as though we had not been separated thousands of miles. We just picked up where we had left off and as though that had been yesterday.

Then I met Marg – Waterstreet that is. For she had recently changed her name after marrying her long-time sweetheart. She was our secretary and we, too, liked each other from the moment that we met. She frequently invited me to the little house that she and Doug rented in Pleasant Valley, a small hamlet true to its name. Both were born in upstate New York. Both were avid nature lovers and we spent many hours exploring the State Parks and forests in and around Duchess County. When I returned to the USA later, I was Auntie Pat to the children. We are still in touch, though not as close as I would have liked. Now Doug is suffering intensely with lung cancer and I think we all feel a little awkward about this. I am reluctant to intrude into their quiet domesticity, although I know that I would be welcome but at what pain and emotional expense.

My third friend was Sadie. She was head of the Social Service Department and we worked together quite intensively. She had had an unhappy marriage and was divorced. She had a delightful daughter who was at this time in college. Sadie loved Italian food and we would treat ourselves at the one Italian restaurant, every now and then. We spent one unforgettable weekend in Rochester for the lilac festival, and another when we visited her property close to Saratoga. Shortly after I returned to Poughkeepsie, Sadie was diagnosed with cancer of the uterus and, despite all medical efforts, succumbed at the early age of fifty-two years.

In the middle of the year, June I think, my classmate Peter moved to his new job at the State Hospital and he was replaced by another English doctor, Margaret Drake. Although I tried to befriend her, I found it very difficult. We just seemed to be totally opposite in our ideas, values and goals. Then one day, it all became very clear. She burst into my room with no announcement very early one morning. I was asleep and awoke to find her trying to climb into bed with me. I rolled over and out of the bed and, despite my naïveté, I realised that 'our Little Drake' was deviant. We continued to be civil to one another, but we had no basis for friendship.

So the year wore on. Since I had no intention of returning to the USA, I spent whatever time and money I had in visiting tourist sites close by, Lake Minewaska, Lake Mohonk, Hyde Park, the Vanderbilt Mansion, as well as New York City and Washington DC. When it was time to leave for home, I felt that I had had a taste of the eastern USA, with its affluence and opulence, its hustle and bustle, and its overwhelming surplus of goods. I had experienced a little of how the other half of the world lived. Yes, it had been a great adventure, but I did not belong there. It wasn't my home. My heart wasn't there. It was time to return to my rightful place. I had no great longing to return to the USA. Life, however, had other plans.

The Return Home

I arrived back in England in July 1953, after five days on the briny aboard the Cunard liner, *Parthia*, in total oblivion and isolated from the real world. My feet were again planted on 'terra firma', with all the sights, sounds and smells familiar to a British subject. We arrived in Liverpool and it would not be long before I was back within the safety and security of that old stone house and amongst the old familiar faces and scenes. Only now did I realise how much I had missed them. Those old adages were true. Familiarity does breed contempt and absence does make the heart grow fonder.

Mother and Dad were waiting and we recognised each other as the liner slowly docked. It would not be long now, before we were together again. Finally, we were a threesome and I knew that

I was home. The solidity of my parents was very apparent, no superficiality, only care from their hearts. Their hugs and kisses let me know, without words, that I was where I should be.

The drive from Liverpool to Matlock took a good three hours. Speed limits were still thirty-five miles an hour and, of course, there was endless chatter as we sped along. We reached Matlock again in late afternoon. What a welcome! The sun was shining, quite a treat in this hilly area where it was so often overcast. Was this a good omen? Just up the hill with its funny name – the Dimple – and I would be truly back where I belonged.

The old stone house was waiting, solid and secure. The garden was aglow with summer blooms, just as it always has been after all those years. What better reassurance could I want that I was back home and in my rightful place? Nothing had changed within those old walls. Everything was in its rightful place. But wait! Where was our little dog? Alas, he had succumbed just after I had left. Could his demise have been connected with my departure, for he really was my pet? My parents tried hard to dissuade me from such thoughts and I tried hard to respond. But there was still a nagging feeling inside of me that just wouldn't go away.

My room was waiting and, it too, showed no change. Great Grandfather's chest glowed familiarly. The bed, with its rosy covers, beckoned invitingly and the book on the bedside table bore promise of happy hours to come. My parents had tactfully left me alone in the old familiar room. Both recognised that I had many thoughts in my head, and that I would need time to think them through. I slowly unpacked and the armoire received the few new clothes I had acquired without any fuss or to do.

Well, here I was, home at last. Lethargy overtook me and I stretched out on the bed with all kinds of thoughts running through my head. How happy I was to be back. A sense of contentment surged through me, but something was missing. Blackie, of course. No matter where I went he had always been at my side. Now his absence must be faced and coped with.

It had been a great year and truly an adventure. I had seen and learned a lot and I had matured as a result. It had been a great thing to do. Dickie had been right. The advantages outweighed the disadvantages. What now, what should I do? What focus did I want for my professional life? Where could I find this? I thought.

Lots of questions needed answers and lots of problems needed solutions. Coming home was not just a simple return to the homeland. Now, for the first time in my life, I really was aware of what life was all about, a mixture of joys and sorrows, headaches and heartaches. Only I can find the solutions, for they somehow must be right for me. That was the hard part, right for me. I knew that all would be solved in due course. The most important thing right now was that I was home with the people I loved and cared about and who loved and cared for me and who would stand by me through the difficult days to come.

Mother always said, 'Where there's a will, there's a way.'

The former would come tomorrow and the way would emerge over the next few weeks. Now, I was just happy to be home and it was time to rejoin my parents and celebrate my homecoming. As I descended the old familiar staircase, the last rays of the sun lit up the last two steps.

Home again in Derbyshire

I slowly adjusted to my English life as each day passed quietly, pleasantly and without excitement. Matlock had not changed. The routine of daily living continued in the same old pattern, up at seven o'clock, a hearty breakfast of bacon, eggs, and toast smothered with home-made marmalade, then off to the day's activities – work or play – home for lunch, then the afternoon women's social activities, tea at four o'clock then the return of the labourers, dinner at six o'clock and then the evening's relaxation. There was no television at this time in my life. We listened to the evening news on the radio, discussed whatever needed to be discussed, then withdraw into our books or played one of the family games – Monopoly, parchesi, dominoes or cards.

At nine o'clock it was news time again, then our bedtime drink – beer for the men and hot cocoa for the women. By ten o'clock, we were all tucked up in our beds and drifting off to sleep. What would tomorrow bring for me? I wondered. I was slowly deciding what I wanted to do with my life and career and how to get myself back on to the right track. This was not easy, for Matlock offered no resources for me and my goals. Slowly, I began to contact my friends, all of whom had continued to stay in the Birmingham area. Slowly, I was assimilated back into the crowd of young medics, all in much the same situation as I was. What should I do, general practice or specialisation? Where should I go, England or overseas? For England was still recovering from World War Two and resources were few and far between. Those who had jobs were not anxious to move on.

As a result of one of our get-togethers, Brenda told me of one available job. A house physician was needed at Little Bromwich Hospital, just outside Birmingham. This was the infectious diseases hospital. Did I really want to go there? I thought. I had been a resident there, during my student years, and had no real need for more experience. Then the phone rang and it was the medical director whom I knew from my previous involvement. He was in need of an experienced physician. The hospital was now studying the new fatal infantile disease as a result of which large numbers of young babies were dying. It was due to infection with B Coli, but we were very ignorant as to how the infection occurred, and the ongoing disease process. He had heard that I was available and would appreciate my help. What could I say? It was like manna from heaven. Of course I wanted to go. What a challenge this would be. So once again I packed my clothes and moved to Little Bromwich Hospital to become involved in one of the few research programmes.

Settling in

Back at Little Brom, as we affectionately called the hospital, all seemed much as before. Little had changed. I was even back in my old room, this time, however with a welcoming floral bouquet to greet me. Many of the senior nurses remembered me. I felt accepted and one of the group. Most of the physicians were newly graduated and didn't know me, but they were friendly and helpful. There was one new sight, a small addition to one of the old wards, built to house the B Coli project. It was clean and fresh and very efficient looking. Each patient had his or her own room, with every essential to hand. What a change it was from the old wards and their rows of beds. Only the assigned nurse and physician were allowed into those rooms and only when gowned and masked. The feeling of isolation in those rooms was awesome but, when one saw the desperate state of each patient, one understood the need for strict hygiene and sterility.

The work was exciting and challenging, but the life-threatening disease and its effects on those tiny human beings was all too overwhelming for the carers. It was one of the greatest challenges for any doctor. To see the response of an infant, initially at death's door then several weeks later discharged to its parents, was both humbling and gratifying. Such success gave rhyme and reason to one's life and a well defined purpose for being. Not all cases were success stories and then one wondered if it was all worth while.

Nothing in the sphere of medicine tugged at the human heart strings more than a desperately sick infant and the urgency of the physical condition was heart-rending. How often we did sweat to get those initial and life-saving, intravenous injections into collapsed infant veins and fluid into dehydrated and almost desiccated bodies. At no time was this performance easy, but what a challenge it was in the middle of the night. Then, after so much struggle, the phone call sometimes came notifying us that Baby Jones's drip had stopped. Worse still, that Baby Smith might have stopped breathing. Yes, those days and nights were filled with emotion and one quickly learned to roll with the punches. We learned to depend on each other for comfort and support.

I don't recall all the details of the research project. Gastro-enteritis was a common disease in infants and young children and was due to many organisms, such as staph, botulism and viruses. Those infants had all the symptoms of a gastro-enteritis infection – vomiting, diarrhoea, and the accompanying body dehydration which could be life-threatening. They did not respond to the tried and trusted remedies at our disposal and the laboratory work was quite erratic and unrevealing. So the search was on. What was the offending organism? It was not one of our known bacteria, and no known antibiotic was effective against it. Was it a virus? As a physician one could only diagnose the condition from the symptoms and provide those little bodies with the essentials for life. The key physicians were the pathologists who were garnering information from autopsies, and bacteriologists who were struggling to identify one organism common to all these cases. The practitioners kept them supplied with essential bodily matter for their experiments. We made these little humans as comfortable as possible and applied appropriate measures to counteract life-threatening situations, living up to our promise to mankind through the Hippocratic oath.

One thing soon became clear to all of us working with those infants. They were in solitary isolation for many hours of each day and this tugged at the heartstrings of the women staff. All the infants needed to be held and rocked, and so we organised a nurturing aspect to the programme. Every infant must receive a certain amount of physical holding and rocking from the nurse in charge of the patient. Yes, we needed more staff, and administration was agreeable to provide this. We were amazed at the positive responses in all those babies and so holding and rocking became essential a part of the therapeutic regime as intravenous injections and medication. As the infants responded to our treatments, the mothers were invited to come as often as possible and provide the contact with their babies.

Whilst my professional life was stimulating, challenging, exciting and at times heart-breaking, my personal life was exciting too, for I had acquired my first car, a convertible Morris Minor, duly christened Clarabelle. How proud I was as I sat behind the wheel! I had really made it now, hadn't I? What more could I want, a good job, friends, a car to go wherever I wanted to go. Yes, I'd come a long way, baby. Weekends were more fun than I could ever remember. I was free to come and go. It was easy to drive home. There was no more waiting for trains and buses. Stratford-on-Avon became a weekly outing and weekend picnics were very much in.

Then came quite a turn of events. I had kept in touch with my American friends, communicating regularly by letter. No startling events were reported, but Peter, my classmate, had decided to specialise in psychiatry. The programme at HRSH had entrapped him and he was fascinated by the mental problems which he was called upon to treat. A course at Columbia University in New York City had opened up a whole new world for him and his ongoing friendship with his British colleagues had led to friendship with the Canadian director of the hospital. He had finally decided to cut the cord and to emigrate to the USA. His parents' distress was not sufficient to throw a damper on his plans. Well, I didn't suppose Peter and I would meet again unless he came over for holidays. Our letters would keep us in touch. Shortly after the letter with Peter's news, I found a rather official letter from the USA awaiting me. It was from HRSH. In essence, the Canadian director was offering me a job, even though he knew that I had had no training or experience in the psychiatric field. There were, he said, plenty of doctors applying for his jobs. Few were proficient in English, and how could you treat psychiatric patients without verbal communication and understanding, he asked.

Why did this letter have to come to me now? I thought. I had just settled back into a happy routine and my life seemed to be moving along in the right direction. Why bother to reply, let alone consider the job as a possibility, but courtesy demanded that I reply in some fashion. As I slowly let idle thought drift through my mind, conflicts of all kinds jumped before my eyes. Of course, I was flattered. Here was someone who barely knew me offering me a job with much security and with excellent training too. How much of this was Peter's doing? As I mulled over the situation, I realised that such a job would never come my way again but did I really want to spend the rest of my life caring for mentally ill patients, and so far from home?

A family conference was called for. What would my parents say? Further inquiries revealed that if I accepted the job, the USA would demand that I declare my intention to become a citizen of that country after five years. Then there was a dilemma. If I did become a citizen I would have to give up my British citizenship. There were no dual citizenships in those days. Well forget it, I thought. I'm British, and British I will stay. Then Dad discovered a way out. I could regain my British citizenship after two years if I maintained an address in the United Kingdom. Well! That would be easy. Nobody was going to take away my home address. That hurdle was over, but it would still be so far away and with little contact with Mother and Dad. Even phone calls were difficult. They had to be booked weeks ahead. Nobody could be reached in a hurry. Mother and Dad were surprisingly encouraging in my returning to the USA.

Conditions in Europe were still very depressed and everyone knew how affluent the Americans were. Perhaps the future did await me there. What could I lose? I should seize the opportunity, for it may not come again. I would come back for the holidays. All my friends supported and encouraged my return. All jokingly said that they would come over for their holidays. What had Dickie's initial comment started now? So, with great ambivalence, I once more packed up and sailed back to New York City in January 1955.

Back in the USA

In January 1955, it was cold in Southampton. As I boarded the Cunard liner reality hit me. For I, too, was now cutting my ties to home, family and friends. What was I doing? Would I be able to make it? Yes! I had friends, but I had little knowledge and experience for what I was about to face. Full of ambivalence, I entered the cabin and met the young woman who would be my cabin mate for the next five days. We were both very much wrapped up in our own thoughts but, as the hours passed, we began to thaw and approach each other. I suggested that we go on deck and watch England fade into the background as the liner pulled away. She preferred to say her goodbyes from below.

As I stood beside the deck rail, my whole life flashed before me and I began to feel a little more cheerful about the whole scene. Nevertheless, I did remind myself that this was not now just an adventure. It was a new chapter in my life and it would unfold and open up only as I made it. Could I do it? I thought. More doubts and more ambivalence assailed me. If only I had one good friend to discuss this with. Then I heard Mother's voice in my mind, Take every opportunity as it comes and make the most of it. Of course, again Mother was right. I would give it my all and see what evolved, I thought. I could always go back home. I knew that I would always be welcome and my own room would be waiting. As we sailed into the open Atlantic, I felt chilled and cold and so I returned to the cabin.

It was dinner time and we were enjoying a delicious meal with two other passengers, both of whom were in good spirits and their chatter and banter carried us along. Then it started. The liner began to rock and roll and pitch and toss. The plates and glasses on the table slid back and forth and were only maintained there by the little wooden edging around the table top which our waiter hurriedly raised. After several more minutes of this, the Captain threw down his napkin and left the dining room. On his return, the motion had ceased and we were once again enjoying our meal. He had told the crew to change course and that did the trick.

Later that night, we were awakened by the pitching and tossing of the liner and a tremendous noise from waves washing over the deck. It sounded as though the waiters were throwing tin trays at each other. Getting up next morning was quite a feat, but one soon learned to let one's body roll with the ship. As we made our way to the dining room we noticed that rope handrails had been attached to every wall and we soon learned how effective they were in helping us to maintain our balance. The Captain announced that we were heading into turbulent seas and that these were so extensive that changing course would not help us, He offered some advice and recommended that we use the rope handrails whenever we left our cabins. This worked well for me, but several travellers lost their balance and suffered fractured arms and legs. In fact, the ship's doctor had never been so busy caring for the passengers. For not only did injuries arise, but a large number of travellers suffered from sea sickness. Again, I was lucky but my cabin mate was confined to her bunk for the next three days and ate nothing but the hard red Washington apples that the nursing staff doled out regularly, as they checked on each patient. I have never eaten one of those hard red apples since. How lucky I was. I made it to every meal and, despite the incessant rocking and rolling, I enjoyed most of the fare that was served. What became readily noticeable was that the number of passengers making it to the dining room became fewer and fewer. Those who did make it showed a camaraderie quite remarkable between strangers. It was interesting for me to recognise how my body responded to the ship's gyrations. I quickly learned that if I rolled in time with the ship's motion, I was in good control.

Of course, this turbulence came to an end. We docked in New York City and that time I was aware of what I needed to do.

Imagine my surprise to be greeted by Peter and another British colleague, my joy at being hustled to the car and driven to Poughkeepsie and HRSH. My little apartment in the resident's building was pleasant and comfortable and I was once again very glad to be back on 'terra firma', but was it the right 'terra firma'? After dinner with the boys, I was glad to sink into bed and sleep came easily. That night passed all too quickly. Now for the new chapter in my life.

I met Dr Alma Freeman in her office, as requested. She was an older grey-haired lady – a Texan – who greeted me warmly, openly and frankly. There was no indication that she would be a difficult boss, but it was very clear that she knew what she wanted and would insist on getting it. She was glad to add yet another British person to her staff and jokingly said that we weren't too difficult to get along with. I was to work on the admissions' unit. Here I would see a wide variety of cases and get a wide variety of experience. Peter would be available to help me and, of course, she was always available, she said. She escorted me to the unit, introduced me to the staff and asked me to stop by her office at half past four. When I did, we discussed my day, my concerns, perceptions, etc. Then she asked me to ride home with her. When we arrived at her residence, a party was obviously in progress. She had sent Peter ahead to organise a little 'welcome to HRSH' party for me and it was thus that I was introduced to the rest of the staff – all Europeans – and all fluent in English.

Because I was a single woman, Dr Freeman invited me frequently to her home. We got to know each other very well. She became my surrogate mother and this helped me through the first year. Our professional experiences had much in common, for Alma's generation were the women pioneers in American medicine. Jobs had been hard to come by, especially in the south. She had become a psychiatrist by chance much like me. She had no regrets, but thought that I would have a wider scope to operate in as women became more accepted in the field. Shortly after I had settled in, Alma pointed out that my pressing need was to acquire a car. Of course, she was right, but how should I go about getting one? I had some money, but not a lot, and my salary was quite meagre.

As luck would have it, she had just bought a new Dodge and her dealer had taken her old one. So we visited him and he still had the car, old in years but young in miles. It was in good working order and he offered me a good deal. So was born another valuable friendship. I was sold on Dodges and always exchanged my old ones for new ones, and always from Mario. I was just as proud of my four-wheeled Alma as I had been of Clarabelle, but now, as I sat behind the wheel, I no longer felt like a carefree adolescent but more like a sedate and sophisticated woman, with a clear purpose and goal to her life. Now I was in a foreign land, committed to a profession. What would be the next challenge? It came soon afterwards. Whilst I could practice temporarily with my British licence, I must take the New York State medical examination. This involved staying in Albany for five days, taking written and oral examinations in all the medical specialties. It was one of the loneliest times of my life, with lots of anxiety and not a soul to share it with. Well, the ordeal ended successfully and I could proudly display my diploma on my office wall.

The days went by, filled with challenges both personal and professional. Winter gave way to spring and spring gave way to summer. My four-wheeled Alma allowed me to explore further and further afield. I could not get enough of the autumn colours. They were so much more vibrant than the English ones and each weekend, my car and I visited the Catskills or Adirondacks.

I was allowed two weeks vacation but I decided to wait and go home for the holidays, Christmas, that is. That was one of the promises I had made to myself and that I intended to keep. That time however, I flew back to England from New York City to London. There were no direct flights at that time. We flew to Halifax in Nova Scotia, refuelled, then to Ireland, refuelled again, and then flew to London. I don't recall all the details of this holiday and I have no photographs to jog my memory, but the keeping of my promise to myself was the most important event of the year, for hadn't I proved, now, that I was able to plan my life, control it to meet my own goals and feel the wonderful satisfaction that this brought. Surely this was what adulthood was all about. If I was right then I had made it. I was now truly grown up.

What is a Psychiatrist?

After I returned from the Christmas holidays, my life fell into a routine and pattern directed by my responsibilities on the wards. Caring for mentally ill patients required the development of new clinical skills. Now I had to understand bizarre and distorted thinking and the skills needed to diagnose physical illness were useless in this situation. Now I had to ask myself, why that seventy year old lawyer from New York City grabbed hold of me whenever I arrived on the ward, and why he did not talk to me about his fears when I invited him into the office? All he expressed were his paranoid feelings and beliefs and though I tried to help him through the techniques that I had been taught, he still did not respond. Why did the thirty year old woman rush from her room whenever she heard the ward door open, throw off her clothes at the feet of whoever entered and sing 'I am now reborn.'

When I left the ward I had much to think about and I leaned heavily on psychoanalytic theories. What did become clear was that all these patients had had troubled lives in their early years. Even with some clear understanding of the psychopathology I was not able to effect much change. Even though most patients responded to their stay with us and were able to go home, it was not long before they were back with the same deviant behaviour and need for protection and safety. Then a new dimension opened up.

With the arrival of Thorazine, psychopharmacology was born. We were now able to medicate mental patients just as we were able to medicate physically ill ones. No longer did we have to restrain uncontrollable patients, nor did we have to watch helplessly as 'crazy' patients thought and acted bizarrely. Now, we felt more like proper doctors using therapeutic skills rather than jailers locking up helpless humans for their protection and safety.

As I slowly gained competence and confidence in this new role, Alma offered me the opportunity to teach. We could all learn together, she said. So I took the three medical students under my wing, and Alma was right. I did learn as I taught, for those youngsters challenged everything that I said. It was summertime, and we spent much free time together, with or without other companions, and my four-wheeled Alma stood us in good stead.

As fall approached, they departed back to their respective schools and I lost touch with them, as my life was about to change.

I was enrolled in the programme at Colombia University. Again, good old Alma carried me back and forth between Poughkeepsie and New York City. We had some tough times as the winter came and there was ice and snow, but we never missed a class. It was here that the biggest event of my life occurred. We were arranged in groups for our clinical sessions. In my group, there was an older woman physician. We seemed to be drawn to each other from the start. We sat together, lunched together and discussed together. She had been divorced after a short marriage to a neurotic husband, after he entered treatment with an analyst. She repeatedly expressed her luck at having her own profession and now her freedom to develop this. Her experience with her husband had convinced her that she should move into psychiatry. So here she was.

In the course of one of our lunches, she asked me what I planned to do with my life. I was quite taken aback, for I had not really thought beyond the next day. I had supposed that I would stay in the state service and, just as the others there, move along as seemed right. Imagine my surprise when she suggested I consider child psychiatry rather than adult psychiatry. This was a new specialty just being born. Clinics had been opened in Chicago, Boston and Philadelphia. She believed that this was to be a whole new answer to psychiatry and who better to be involved than women doctors? If we could identify deviancy in childhood, could we not intervene and prevent later illness? Now we were embarking on psychopharmacology. What possibilities might just be round the corner? My friend had opened up a whole new world of ideas and I couldn't wait to get back and discuss all this with Alma. She, too, saw much logic in it and it made sense in terms of her vast clinical experience. For me, it was the way to go. I was young, life was ahead of me.

'Yes! Go to Philadelphia and see for yourself what is going on,' she said.

Again what could I lose? After many phone calls to a Dr John Rose at the Child Guidance Clinic, I was given an appointment to meet with him. I arrived at the interview drenched and looking like a drowned rat, for I had had to park a dozen blocks from the clinic and, as I started to walk there, the rain came and was suddenly a deluge. I had no umbrella and no shelter and time was getting closer and closer to the appointment.

Doctor Rose appeared not to notice my dishevelled state. We talked about my experiences, my interests, my relationships with others and then out of the blue he asked, 'What behaviour in children do you dislike most?'

I was totally taken aback but, after struggling with my thoughts and my minimal experience with children, I replied as best I could.

'I can't stand bullies.'

It was only years later that I understood the method in his madness, for I had queued him into my own unconscious hang-ups. He nodded in dismissal and his secretary said that they would be in touch. Well, that was the end of that, I thought. That interview had been a new experience for me. I had never met anyone so distant and so unrelated as Dr Rose. As I drove back to Poughkeepsie, I said goodbye to Philadelphia and didn't expect to see that city again. As it turned out, I had been quite wrong about Dr Rose. He had been very well tuned in to me. Can you believe that I arrived in Philadelphia to become part of his research team on 1 January 1957? At that time, I had no idea that my professional life was settled, that I was on the right track and that that was the beginning of my life's work. Philadelphia was to become my home for the next forty years.

The Philadelphia Story, 1957 to 1998

Philadelphia

As I settled into my first floor, one roomed apartment in a classical Philadelphia Brownstone building on Pine Street, Dickie's face flashed before me and, in my mind, I heard the words, What do you have to lose? Well, the adventure had moved to a commitment to a new homeland and a career in a profession that was just being born. If I wanted to be romantic, it sounded like a whole new life was before me, just like the pioneers of a generation ago. Let's be realistic! What did I lose? In all honesty, not much. My homeland was still there, across a mighty ocean, but still easily accessible. My family and friends were there and very much in contact. Letters crossed the briny frequently. I missed those spontaneous outings and get-togethers but then those would happen here with the new friends that I was making.

I guessed that the question really was, 'What had I gained?' First, it was fair to say that I had grown up. I now had better self-awareness, I was goal oriented and developing myself both personally and professionally. I was independent. I could support myself, run a car and indulge myself modestly. I had made new friends. How true they were would only become clear as life went on. I had broadened my outlook with travel and by experimenting with all kinds of new foods and I think I now evaluated situations more sensibly and practically. Yes, I had gained a lot in the past three years, but not much materially. My meagre apartment, with its meagre possessions, did not suggest a successful professional. How had my classmates fared in their English life style? Those I know had married the fellows that they dated in medical school. They were settled and their life was purposeful. Most had material things and most had some form of debt, a mortgage or car payments. I had no debt, but then I had no need for extraneous belongings. Again, Mother's voice reminded me that independence was the name of the game and my career was the key to that.

Now it was 1 January 1957, it was another new beginning. Although I did not know it, it was to be the beginning of the direction and purpose of my future life. On 2 January 1957, I arrived at the clinic early, and was greeted by James, the janitor. Yes, everyone would come in today, just wait here in the lobby, he told me. Suddenly, the door was thrown open and a huge man of about six feet four inches, with a heavy overcoat and fedora, burst through out of the bitter cold. He looked quite menacing, but he smiled, greeted me cheerfully and said that everyone would be there at nine o'clock. Goodness, I was early, I thought. There were still ten minutes to go. He was right. Everyone reassembled after the holiday weekend and I was led to my office, then introduced to my supervisor, Dr Donald Ross, a Canadian. He gave me the low-down on the clinic and the way that we would work and a ten page pamphlet to read. As I opened this later, I was impressed by the opening lines – 'Some of us are here to teach, but we are all here to learn.' Isn't that what Alma had said?

My routine was highly academic. I was to learn how to diagnose emotional disturbance in children and learn how to treat the condition. Lectures had a specific foci on emotional disturbance, psychopathology, symptoms and needs. Nobody could define emotional disturbance for me. The closest I could come to an answer to my question, 'What is ED?', was that those children do not act appropriately for their age and can be difficult to control. Along with the lectures, I was given a caseload of patients – six in all as I recall – who had been diagnosed by my supervisor. It was my responsibility to work with the child, his family and school, when possible, under Dr Ross's supervision. This meant that every step was worked out before I saw the child, and implemented in the clinical setting, only when I was clear as to why this was to be. The year would be one of the most difficult of my career. I remembered my graduation promise – better to go down in the swirling foam than in the sluggish delta. Well, here was the swirling foam.

Philadelphia Child Guidance Clinic

Here I was, settling in at the Child Guidance Clinic. Three other

'Fellows' who had arrived in September were already well into the programme and its course. They were Ora Smith, a Canadian physician, Marvin Weiner, a PhD in psychology from New York City and Al Shire, also a PhD in psychology, from New Jersey. Al was married and his wife and infant son were with him. They, too, had Brownstone apartments either on Pine or Spruce Street, as did several of the clinic social work staff. So I became a member of this Inner City group. We worked hard and spent many of our leisure hours together.

Again the pattern was repeating itself. I had a stimulating and challenging job and a pleasant social group. I quickly learned that child psychiatry involved only a very small professional group. There were four thousand trained professionals to serve the whole of the USA. As I got to know those people, another odd coincidence occurred. Ora had trained at the University of Dalhousie in Halifax, Nova Scotia and had graduated one year later than I had. We had been taught pathology by the same doctor – Bill Abbyss – who had emigrated to Dalhousie in July, after my pathology course at Birmingham. We then learned that Bill was now practising in Wilmington, Delaware. We contacted him and found that he was in the process of divorcing his wife, because she refused to live in America and had returned to England to live. Bill and I became very good friends and I believe we would have finally married, but my life became hectic and he ran into difficulties with the divorce.

January passed quickly and on 1 February, another Fellow joined us at the clinic. This time, it was another woman physician from the Ukraine. Her name was Wira Trigos. As the year progressed, Wira and I were thrown together and we became real buddies. She had recently married and she and her husband, an adult psychiatrist, were living in Princeton, New Jersey. What a trip she had every day, but when her husband's residency ended, he moved to Friend's Hospital in Philadelphia and they moved to their first house in Secane. Now they, too, became members of our social group. As 1957 came to its close, we all evaluated our progress as child psychiatrists. We had come a long way but we still had far to go.

Then, in the New Year, Wira and I – not the men – were

summoned to Dr Rose's office. He was hoping to develop a research project – later named the Maternal Attitudes Study. We were to be key figures in helping him to develop this project. We were to meet with the chief physician of the Antenatal Clinic at Pennsylvania Hospital and arrange to talk to the pregnant women registered there. The obstetrician was somewhat sceptical but he was at least tolerant. His experience had confirmed that the population of Inner City black mothers-to-be were not easy to communicate with, but he would support our efforts and he agreed that every woman registered at the clinic would be given the option to talk to us.

'What should we talk about?' we asked Dr Rose.

'Her perception of this whole new experience that she is facing,' he replied. 'Her pregnancy, her labour, and her impending motherhood.'

Little was known of the latter. Some research had been published by Ackerman and Helen Deutch, but most of what the average women knew and understood about this important developmental stage was passed down within families from mother to daughter and mixed in with old wives' tales. Most of the women accepted this opportunity to talk and this convinced us that we were on to a pressing need. Wira and I had more interviews arranged than we had ever envisaged or thought possible.

All our interviews were taped. Since neither Wira nor I were mothers, we had many questions about our lack of knowledge. This stood us in good stead, for we were not able to interject our knowledge and deflect the mother-to-be's thinking and responses. Anyway, we were there to listen to what was being said. We were not there to interpret it to our clients. Each day we raced back to the clinic, settled in Dr Rose's office and listened avidly with him to our conversations. We were all learning together. Imagine how proud we were when Dr Rose lauded our efforts. Never had such personal data been revealed. What a three months that was! We lived and breathed interviews. We were staying until late hours at the clinic and arriving as early as seven o'clock and then trudging down to the clinic for more grist for the mill.

At the end of that three months, Dr Rose took samples of our tapes to Washington and the National Institute of Mental Health.

The people there were impressed with our data and Dr Rose's hypothesis for the project. Funding was granted and the Maternal Attitudes Study was born. As we continued gaining experience, we began to see that a standardised semi-structured interview could be developed and used, and slowly the Maternal Attitudes Study was extended to other academic centres and the National Perinatal Project was born, involving all the major university medical schools.

In essence, mothers-to-be were interviewed during their pregnancy. We soon found that the ideal time was around the fifth month after foetal movements had occurred, making the mother-to-be aware of another human being within them. For it was this realisation that promoted their thinking and planning as to what was to come, and how they were going to cope with it and how this new arrival would affect their lives.

From the data gathered in these interviews, we became aware that we had information from which we could predict the outcome of the pregnancy, the type of labour that the mother-to-be would experience and, furthermore, the type of child-rearing practices that the new mother would use. Correlating the mother's behaviour with child development, Dr Rose utilised a quadrant analysis, which defined infant behaviour that would predominate. In those mother–infant relationships where caring and rearing practices were absent, distorted or unrelated to the infant's needs, nurturant or developmental, deviant behaviour occurred in the infant – often as early as the first year. The project was funded for us to follow these infants every four months for the first year and then, regularly, until the age of seven years. Thus, we had constant information as to how our predictions were holding up.

As we gained more and more experience, we began to see that our Maternal Attitudes Study could be used for early identification of impending deviant motherhood and infant development. Would this give us an opportunity for early intervention? We also came to realise that the Maternal Attitudes Study interview could be adapted into a more extensive one, for diagnostic and evaluative processes in child psychiatry. What a hectic time this was! But wasn't my friend at Columbia right? Yes! I had made the right decision and I had nothing to lose. I must just keep my nose to the grindstone and who knows what would occur. I had come a long, long way as a result of those few words issued by Dickie Gillespie, 'Go to America, what do you have to lose?' What a shame that he never knew what he had done for my career.

Another Challenge

During the year, Marga came to visit me in Philadelphia, on her way back home to Germany. She had had excellent training at the University in Chicago and felt that she was now very able to move into private practise in her homeland, where she was needed by her ageing parents. A position had opened up in Bad Reichenhall and she was to be the junior partner in a flourishing practice. Before she left, she insisted on scrubbing my beige rug. What a gesture! What she did not realise was that it was August – hot and humid – and it took weeks for that rug to dry, despite our hanging it over the shower curtain rod, to say nothing of the inconvenience to taking a shower. We later had many good laughs over that episode!

As we said goodbye, we promised to keep in touch and we are still fulfilling that promise. The next time that we met – I think five years later – I was a married woman and she enjoyed meeting my husband and child. Meanwhile the Maternal Attitudes Study research was the focus of my life. Others were working in the field of early childhood development – Bakwin, Harlow with his monkeys, Goldfarb, Lebovici in France, Ainsworth, Province and Lipson. All had identified emotional deprivation, i.e. lack of physical and emotional togetherness between mother and infant, as the precursor of deviant child development.

Bowlby claimed that the beginnings of mental health and ill health were to be found in the infant's relationship with the mother. But what was the basis of this relationship? Our data seemed to indicate that mother and infant must bond if normal development was to follow. This seemed to confirm Bowlby's own notion that deprivation of attachment between mother and infant affected personality development adversely. As our data accumulated, Dr Rose gave me the responsibility of writing up our project and the results that we were seeing. So my first paper was born and published in *Child Welfare* in July 1965. Now the question was, could we use our new-found knowledge for early intervention and possible prevention of mental illness? How could we use it? Child psychiatrists had no access to babies and infants but paediatricians did. Now the next challenge arose. Could we work with paediatricians, imbue them with our knowledge and include it in their clinical practice?

I was the one chosen for this task. Dr Rose had established a close working relationship with the head of a department known as Psychological Paediatrics at the Children's Hospital. A meeting was called, attended by Dr Rose, Dr Shuford and his Fellow, Dr Bayley and me. They all seemed somewhat leery of a woman physician. They were interested in the ideas, but left mumbling something about funding. After they had left, Dr Rose, for the first time since I had known him, was supportive and reassuring and said that it would all work out and we would probably begin to work together in the New Year.

'Great!', I said.

Later that evening, I realised that my two year fellowship would be over at the end of December and another vital decision would have to be made, to stay at Philadelphia Child Guidance Clinic, or move out into the wide, wide world. Again the decision was made for me. Chet Deates, the director of the Wilmington Child Guidance Clinic was anxious for me to join his staff and relieve him of some clinical responsibilities and allow him time for administrative work. He also hoped to incorporate some of our new ideas into his practices. So I worked in Wilmington for two days and in Philadelphia for three days each week. I was still friendly with Bill Abbyss and I moved into Kynlyn Apartments in the suburbs of Wilmington. We continued to meet and enjoy each other's company until his wife returned to finalise their divorce. W agreed to discontinue our meetings, so as not to interfere with these proceedings. Meanwhile, the project with the paediatrics in Philadelphia was about to start and my life once again reverted to intense involvement and took on a new direction.

2 January 1960

It was lunch time on 2 January 1960 and I was munching with a group of staff members in the hospital coffee shop.

A voice from behind me said, 'Hey, you're going to be my child psychiatrist.' I turned to confront the Director of Psychological Paediatrics.

My response was 'Oh, and since when? Nobody has told me so.'

It was true and I was soon summoned to Dr Ross's office, where the news was confirmed. Prior to my starting in this new role, the Child Guidance Clinic alumnae meeting was to be held, and guess what! I was elected to present a case together with Dr Shuford using our new hypotheses and ideas. This meant collaboration on a daily basis – sometimes during clinic hours – sometimes after clinic hours, when we would grab a bite to eat in the coffee shop, as we discussed how best to do the job.

The evening of the meeting arrived. I was tense and anxious. This was the first time that I had spoken before a large group of colleagues – mostly older and much wiser and more experienced than I was. How would they respond? Who would bale me out? I was consoling myself that Dr Shuford was more experienced and would rise to the occasion when who should enter the room but the man himself. From all appearances, he was more scared than I was. I don't recall any details of the meeting and so I guess all went well. I would have been made aware if it had not. Anyway, this was the beginning of the new challenge – working with paediatricians – a challenge that was to last for the next forty years.

The programme started. I was to work alongside Dr Bayley – Joe, as he later came to be known – in the neonatal clinic. We got along well for he was a good-natured, easy going southerner. At our weekly sessions with Dr Ross and Hank, we were subjected to little criticism and, after six months, I was asked to write up my impressions of this experience. Joe was similarly requested and we all met with the professor of paediatrics. He was suitably impressed and our ideas were incorporated into the resident's training. I returned to my clinical responsibilities and my social life became quite hectic. Joe and I had been drawn to each other and he had invited me out on several dates. The most impressive was to an army navy game, where we were treated like royalty for the captain of the navy team had been a shipmate of Joe's during the war.

Then Dr Shuford called to invite me to the opera. He had two tickets to *La Bohème* and asked if I would join him for dinner and the show. The old question reared its head. What did I have to lose? I loved Puccini and it was a pleasant evening and, as we said goodnight, I thought that was the end of that, but not so. He kept inviting me for other dates. It all became too much. Then he started inviting Joe to join us and we became a threesome, until I suggested that he include one of the social workers whom we all liked. As we became a foursome, Bertha, who was older and wiser than I was, began to see what was happening, and she was right. For after an evening of Gilbert and Sullivan at Longwood Gardens, it was arranged that Joe take Bertha home and Dr Shuford should take me back to Wilmington. He asked to come into the apartment and then told me that he liked me and would like to date me. I was flabbergasted. That was the first indication of any romantic aspect to our relationship. I can't remember what I replied, but I did indicate that I was not looking for an intimate relationship, although I liked him as a friend. Our relationship continued in that vein, at least for the next few months.

Marriage and Motherhood

The Axe Falls

Puccini won and, after a short courtship, we were quietly married on 19 August 1961, witnessed by a select group of the Shuford family and mutual friends.

'Now,' said Hank, 'you are my wife as well as my child psychiatrist.'

Not only had I acquired a husband, but also his two children, Mary, aged ten, and Jim, aged seven years. After the wedding reception, the guests dispersed, the children and Martha, their carer, set off for a week on a farm and we slowly locked up the house and set off for our honeymoon – a week touring eastern Canada.

I was thirty-six and he was forty, and we frequently joked, 'Well, life begins at forty, so let's get on with it.' Well, a different life began for me and what a challenge it was to be. I was emotionally ready to settle down into some kind of domesticity, and I very much wanted a child of my own. For my child would be the human being to keep the Johnson family well and alive. For my sister and her husband had let the family know that they had opted to not have offspring. So it was up to me. My idea of domesticity was based on my parent's life style, but these ideas were soon to change.

Our first pressing need was immediately evident – a larger house with room for privacy and separation as well as togetherness. We looked at suburban house after suburban house and found nothing that appealed to us. Then one wet and miserable Sunday afternoon in February, we found it.

We looked at each other after walking through and said unanimously, 'That's it.'

It became ours. Now we could let our old lives and individual interests go and start to build a life together. We were married, committed and anxious to settle into our own haven with the children. I had just learned that I was pregnant. What a hectic year, selling a house and buying another one and the children changing schools, but we were settled into our home before our child was born on 12 August 1962. This, too, like most of the experiences in my life, was another challenge. The pregnancy had been uncomplicated but the delivery made little headway. The nursing staff, as usual, blamed me, but not for long, as foetal distress became evident and I was rushed to the operating room and a Caesarian section was performed, but what a joy. I had a big bouncing girl, weighing eight pounds twelve ounces. All went well post-natally and I returned with our baby to our new home on the tenth day. The older children had decorated the hallway with balloons and flowers and were both excited and awed by the precious bundle that I carried into her home. Just as in all families, the new arrival enforced necessary changes and, at times, these were hard on all of us, but more so on the other children especially when Martha decided that she did not want to be carer to a new infant. She had had her fill of babies, she said. I was still on the staff at the Child Guidance Clinic and, despite their knowledge of early infancy and its needs, there was great pressure for me to return to the office. After much searching, we found Elizabeth, a kind, warm-hearted and experienced Afro-American lady to care for our infant Esther and the older children whilst I was away. Elizabeth became one of us and she stayed with us in varying capacities until she died twenty-one years later.

We Must Practice What We Preach

'Wifehood and motherhood all in one year,' said my friend Bertha. 'That's biting off more than you can chew.'

Yes, but I'm a late starter, I consoled myself, when life got a little choppy. Remember what Dad said, prioritise when things get out of hand. It was not so easy when there were four people dependent on me. Hank and I commuted to Philadelphia together daily, so we had time to ourselves to talk or just enjoy each other's company as the need arose. We always tried to have one evening a week out by ourselves, usually Friday, as a fitting end to a hectic week and so that we could be with the children at the weekends.

When we were out, I always made sure that there was an exciting addition to the children's evening.

Elizabeth always had an orderly house for me to return to after a busy day. The children's physical needs were extra well cared for, but I soon realised how needy they were for adult attention and approval. It was easy for me to include Mary into my life. She enjoyed being part of all the feminine activities, and she loved to shop, but I had great difficulty finding togetherness with Jim. Even his father could not get close to him for he showed little interest in sports or other masculine activities. He spent hours watching dramatic television programmes, and so we tried to share some of the artistic side of life. My efforts to reach his heart through his stomach had some effect, as the menu included hot dogs, hamburgers and Kentucky fried chicken.

Esther was a socially outgoing infant. Even in the newborn nursery, she attracted attention with her sparkling eyes. She loved to be held and cuddled and played with. When she was five months old Jim's cat, Rebbie, was killed on the highway and we replaced the cat with a Sheltie pup called Prince. Our infant enjoyed this new addition more than any of us, and they quickly became inseparable. For me, it was like having twins, or so I supposed. I always knew where the human infant was, but I wasn't always sure where the canine could be found, although he was never far away, especially if Esther had a cookie which she quickly learned to use as bait.

As parents, Hank and I had very different ideas about raising children. His southern background encouraged closeness and dependency. My upbringing encouraged caring and independence. When we couldn't agree on what was needed, I would revert to our research study data, but that seldom helped and we struggled with our differences for the rest of our lives. We spent much time with the children. I wanted a happy, trusting, well knit family. Such does not happen overnight and, as the children reached adolescence, our differences and resolutions became harder and harder to take. For my life after marriage was a whole new and alien experience. Nobody I knew had married a divorcee and nobody I knew had acquired a family. Just as I had grown professionally, now I had to grow personally.

My greatest dilemma was trying to solve the problems with the knowledge I had learned from my own stable family. Could these work in this hodgepodge family situation? Yes, they would and could provided that both parents defined, accepted, supported and enforced them together, but nobody could judge the guilt and shame and the sense of failure toward the children when marriages failed and remarriage occurred. Nobody could know the agony experienced by the children and their fear that it was all their fault. This became a trap for the new members trying to develop another primary family. How could they believe, trust in, and be loyal to their elders? Why would this time work any better than the one before? No wonder our society was becoming chaotic and disordered for nobody played by the same rules of life. Yet all would agree that nobody could win a soccer or hockey game, if the team did not stick to the rules. Despite the stress, the conflicts and the difficulties, I did insist on routine, structure and stability in our daily lives and the children blossomed forth. All loved school and did well. All made friends and no one was noticeably affected by the sixties and the drug using peers. Elizabeth followed my orders and deviated only with my permission.

Mealtimes were family times in our house and it was there that we learned about each other's activities, thoughts and ideas. I tried to interject fun and jokes to lighten what could have been rather sombre times and usually the children responded. We tried to encourage responsibility by having the young ones help with the chores and with planning menus, cooking and serving. Once all was cleaned and neat, we settled down with or without the children, and we encouraged quiet and relaxing activities in preparation for sleep and readiness for the next day. So life went on and the years passed.

The Holidays

Our English summer sojourns started when Esther was two years old. My parents and family had not met my new family and so we arranged for Elizabeth, Mary and Bill to be with us too. What excitement there was in just getting to England on that overnight flight and the welcome that we received on arrival. There were lots of mixed feelings on everyone's part – except on the part of Esther, who celebrated her second birthday amidst her doting relatives. Father and Mother were grandparents, something that they had become resigned to not be, since Sis and Eric had told them of their wish to not procreate, and marriage did not seem imminent in my life. Well, it had happened and Dad was one of the happiest men in the world. Now, the family would go on, even if the name didn't. This was the only year my stepchildren visited with us. It was as important for them to know their mother and her family, and so they headed south as we went east.

I looked forward to my yearly trips home, but what confusion this always created. Can you imagine packing sweaters when it was ninety degrees plus outside and extra humidity? Those three weeks in my homeland always brought me back to earth, increased my faith in humanity and restored my own self-confidence. Those old values were true and worth fighting for. Have the courage of your convictions, rang in my head whenever I was in doubt. Most of all, those three weeks brought Mother and I close. It was on my fortieth birthday that we became as one and I felt that I had finally joined that league of women who always seemed not available to me. Now I was experiencing all those challenges that face every woman, as wife and mother, and Mother had coped with these challenges too. Our quiet discussions helped me see my life more objectively and enabled me to see those challenges with a clearer perspective. Yes, life continued to teach us, but we had to be willing to learn.

As Esther moved into childhood, we needed to find interesting activities for her to enjoy beside the inevitable visiting and travelling. On her sixth birthday, Mother and Dad settled us in the car and they drove us to Tansley, a nearby village. We stopped at a little farm. We were obviously expected and we were led out to the stables. Here was a little pony, ready and waiting for Esther. She was thrilled. Dad had arranged it all. We came back every day, whilst we were in Matlock. Hank also enjoyed the activity and so started Esther's love of riding which lasted into her high school years. As soon as we returned to the USA, we located a riding school in the suburbs, owned and run by a British family, and Esther soon became the proud owner of a small mare, whose name escapes me now. This was a demanding hobby. She rode at weekends and one day midweek and, after the lesson it was her responsibility to care of the animal and ensure that she was settled comfortably in her stall. I was the chauffeur and was glad when we had the opportunity to pool cars with another family. It was a wonderful hobby for Esther. Not only did it encourage her love of nature but she became an accomplished rider and won many ribbons in the local shows. Needless to say, I had some pretty tense moments when she started to learn to jump the horse, all unnecessary, of course, but mothers cannot help being mothers.

Every Thanksgiving morning we rose with the lark and drove to the stable, readied the mare and then drove to join the Radnor Hunt. Esther and her peers followed the hounds on their horses. We followed in the car. When the fox had been run to earth, we all joined the huntsmen in their traditional celebration of drinking from the stirrup cup. Then we went back home to catch our breath and enjoy a traditional Thanksgiving dinner, with or without family and friends.

As Christmas approached again, there was more excitement. Now it was time to bring home our Yuletide tree. Hank and the children would select and cut the tree. I would be waiting with a meal, which was swallowed quickly, for cutting and lugging that tree gave everyone a good appetite. Then came the trimming and we would include friends whenever possible.

We always had two Christmas celebrations. One just before the actual day when we all celebrated together and one on the day itself, with just the three of us. Always on this day we talked to Mother and Dad over the phone, a call which had been booked weeks beforehand. As the years passed, and the children scattered, Mother, Sis and Eric began to visit at this time and once again my family was reunited for the holidays. The Europeans were always amazed at the glamour and extravagances and our overindulgence at this season. Christmas in England still was considered a religious holiday and the festivities were symbolic of the religious ceremony. I remember the symbolism of all the Christmas tree ornaments, but this seemed so trite here in this overabundant land. Those Christmas get-togethers continued for many years and long after Mother and Eric had left us and even now, we shared the spirit of the moment even if not on the traditional day. So the years passed and life went on.

The In-laws

Just as we kept close ties with the distaff side of the families so too did we attempt to keep related to Hank's large family. This was not so easy. He was one of seven children and his siblings were scattered around the south. Charles, who travelled extensively for his company, stopped with us when he was in our area and later his son Chuck became an intimate member of our family during his college years at Haverford. This was the one family that I felt close to and part of this was because Alice, Charles's wife, and I had much in common. She, too, had been a professional woman and her ideas and values were akin to mine, for she had grown up in Kansas.

The annual family reunion was the avenue for togetherness. Since one of the sisters had a summer home on Fripp Island, this was the chosen site for the gathering. What a mêlée those days were! I remember as many as forty-five family members gathering one year. What a commotion and what a to do there was. It was impossible to enjoy a quiet moment with just one person, for there was always someone pushing past, or interrupting or yelling across the room. Even outdoors it was no better. If someone had something to say it had to be said. Was this the way in large families? I asked myself. It was alien to me, for shouting and yelling and interrupting were no-nos in my family. There was time for all of us – we were only four. I found this nerve-racking and tried to hide from it all.

The first reunion that I attended was alcohol free in deference to the oldest brother and leader of the clan. How to relieve the tension that settled in one's head and body, among such noise and confusion, I wondered. How am I going to survive without some form of tranquilliser? I thought. Fripp Island was quite isolated but I made some excuse to go to the nearest town, Beaufort, and I smuggled a bottle of Scotch back to our room and retired for a quiet and soothing drink whenever the turmoil got to be too much. I don't think I was the only culprit. For the next time that we attended one of these reunions, the oldest grandchild, Dick, now in his late thirties, arranged for punches to be served, one laced and one non-alcoholic. At subsequent affairs, wine was served with dinner.

My in-laws were a nice group and I was accepted into the family, without hesitation. What I quickly learned was that in no way could I fit into the southern life style. The rigidity, the narrow-mindedness, the arrogance of the men and subjugation of the women were not for me, or dependency – when would I expect my dinner partner to order for me without some discussion? I felt stifled and demeaned. I was so glad to be on the way back to our northern home.

When I expressed these feelings to Hank, his response was, 'Why do you think I went north?'

So he had felt the oppression too, after freedom in the navy, but those old attitudes stuck with him for as long as I knew him. Again, Mother had been right – get independent. Now all these years later, I see some of the great-grandchildren in this family striving to find some semblance of this for themselves, but few were supported by their parents. Slowly it will come, for life goes on.

Sorrows and Sadness

It was October 1969. We had settled back into our routine after our English holiday when the phone rang. Mother, very perturbed, was calling to say that Dad had had a heart attack but that he was holding his own and refused to go to hospital. We dropped everything, got the plane that evening and were home in Matlock as soon as it was possible. We met the family physician when he visited the next day. He was new to the practice and had replaced old Dr Sparks. All was going well, he said, but Dad needed much encouragement to stay in bed and rest for the prescribed ten days. I was determined to stay with my parents until after that critical tenth day. If Dad survived that, all would be well. Hank returned home for there was little that he could do except watch and wait and this was not his forte.

Again Mother and I were given the opportunity for closeness. We seemed to be moving closer and closer. Dad survived the dreaded day and, after he was up and about, I returned to the

USA. Just before I left Mother, drew me to one side and said, 'Always remember that your room is ready and waiting, if ever you should need it.'

In the heat of the moment I thanked her but later, on the plane, I wondered what she was hinting. I don't know, so I gave up. I had so much else on my mind.

On our next trip over, in summer 1970, Dad seemed to be his old self, full of energy and enthusiasm but when I said goodbye and hugged him, I felt his physical frailty and that night in the airport motel, I cried for the first time in my married life. I needed a little comfort, but only Esther offered me any. I realised that Dad's life was on the wane and so I wasn't too surprised when the call came in October. Dad had passed on. He had risen from the table, after enjoying his usual breakfast of eggs and bacon, and had collapsed onto the floor, dead.

Again, we raced home and the few family members had gathered at Kelvin Grove, the saddest reunion that house had witnessed in my lifetime, but where were Sis and Eric? They were touring in France. Despite police attempts to locate them we had heard nothing from them. Then the next day, there they were. They had heard their name over the car radio, had checked in with the local police and headed straight for home. So we said goodbye to Dad.

Dad's demise created a real problem for Mother, who did not want to live alone. A new life started for all of us. Mother would stay with us in the USA for six months and with Sis and Eric in their home in Eastbourne for the rest of the year. She sold the old family home to a local dentist, with whom Sis maintained professional relationship for several years to come. Our new life worked well for all of us. It kept our little family together. It would have been so easy to drift apart, just because of the distances. This togetherness continued for the next eight years.

In 1978, Hank and I went to England to be with Mother following her hip replacement. She was back home and all was going well but that night, she had pains in her chest and was hospitalised the next day for a pulmonary embolism. She responded to all the treatment poorly and I think that she had given up. She had said several times that it was time to go. On the fifth day, whilst I was visiting in the intensive care unit, she became very agitated and told me that it was the end. She begged me to go home and get on with my own life. She said that I deserved to be happy. Reluctantly, I left her after a very casual kiss. We were a solemn group that evening. I went early to bed. Yes, again Mother was right! The hospital called at two o'clock in the morning. She had left us on my fifty-fourth birthday. What was it about that date? My favourite aunt had died on the day before, five years ago and Eric later died one day after my birthday five years later. We buried her with Dad, as they had requested and, at the end of the burial service, I felt like an orphan. Again, I felt that ambivalence. I wanted to go home and I wanted to stay at home. Well, no matter what, sunshine or rain, life still went on.

The Prime of Life

Another Professional Challenge

Yes! life did go on and, as Hank constantly reminded me, I now had my own family and the responsibilities that this entailed. I also had my career. Shortly after our marriage, Dr Rose had died and I did not want to stay at the Child Guidance Centre under its new director. Again, Fate rescued me. Dr Phylis Schaefer, an older woman child psychiatrist, invited me to join her in her efforts to establish a mental health programme within the Philadelphia school system. This was a whole new concept for mental health workers. Others across the country were struggling with it, too.

Why did so many inner city children have trouble in school? If we could understand why, then we could perhaps help. We decided to utilise the data and formats from the Maternal Attitudes Study and to determine if there was any correlation between the mother and child relationship and the child's learning. For we were impressed by the fact that most of the children with learning problems had the intellectual ability to learn. What was stopping them? Were racial issues at the root of it? Several teachers told us that they could predict problems in first graders and these predictions were confirmed by third grade. What clued them in? Some thought that it was the child's developmental levels. So we began to interview the mothers as well as to evaluate the children and, as in the Maternal Attitudes Study, to correlate maternal attitudes and caring practices with the child's developmental levels and academic performance.

At this time, the Federal government had passed PL94 142. Every school district was to provide special education programmes for those handicapped children, who fell within the category of ED – emotional disturbance. We were really in business and special education classes were organised in every district throughout the city. Shortly after this, Dr Schaefer became ill and died rather suddenly from cancer. Now, I was left holding the bag. As I worked intensively with the teachers and school counsellors the programme developed. My second paper was written and published. It was entitled, 'A School Mental Health Programme' published in *Mental Health*, volume 52, in 1968.

The city programme developed by leaps and bounds and I needed help. Who could help me? Of course, only Wira. She had deserted her professional life for motherhood five years ago. Her daughter was now five and on her way to kindergarten. Wira did not let me down. She responded to my need and, even though we worked together, we needed more and more help. I approached our local regional council – the organisation to which all child psychiatrists belonged – and enlisted a group of twelve well trained professionals, all avid and eager to be included in this new dimension of child psychiatry.

The professors of psychiatry at the five universities in Philadelphia were impressed with the programme and we arranged for their child psychiatric residents to be included in the programme. Yes, Dickie! I've really made it, I said to myself. I am the director of the programme, I have twelve excellent staff, residents in training and what's more an associate professorship from Jefferson University.

Life again was hectic. It went on and went on. More papers were written. Some were presented orally and some were published. In the spring of 1983, I presented one of these papers – entitled Prediction and Outcome for Families and Infants at risk for Mental Disorder – to the Second World Congress of Infant Psychiatry in Cannes, France. It read as follows:

> The infants born into The Maternal Attitudes Study were part of the population of the National Project and were followed intensively from birth to seven years of age. A report by Spivak of a twelve year follow up study of students in the Philadelphia School System had confirmed our clinical impression that many youth were highly vulnerable and at risk. Larger and larger numbers of children – five and six year olds – with severe development deficits from severely dysfunctional families were constantly referred to the Child Psychiatric Services to determine what educational and therapeutic interventive efforts were

needed.

In the city of Philadelphia, we have had available to us extensive data on approximately five thousand students, evaluated by the Philadelphia Collaborative Perinatal Project from birth to seven years, who have been or are currently in the public school system.

In collaboration with our research colleagues, we have reviewed this data for one specific group of students – approximately one hundred and fifty – identified through the Office of Psychiatric Services as having developmental deficits of such severity as to interfere with academic progress and/or socialisation skills.

Our goal was to determine what risk factors, if any, occurred uniformly within this group and if each could be validly utilised to identify other students at the time of school entrance.

What fun we had! The paper was accepted but, best of all, we shared it all with friends and family. Joe Bayley and Sally Tollinger flew over with us. Sis and Eric drove from England to join us and, best of all, Marga and her two friends drove from Bertchesgarden, where she was now the obstetric and gynaecology physician for that city. Everyone enjoyed that little holiday. We returned home for Easter and, shortly after the holiday, Hank and I flew to Seattle to meet up with a group of child psychiatrists. Under the auspices of 'People to People' we went to visit China, to determine what, if anything, our small specialty had to offer this ancient culture and its children.

China

A letter arrived, offering a trip to China with the Academy of Child Psychiatrists. I wanted to go.

'No, don't go there,' said Hank. Something inside me kept telling me I needed to go. What's the matter with me? I wondered. Then there flashed before my eyes a picture of long ago. I was ten years old. Walking on the streets in Matlock was a lady who was obviously not one of us. It was very unusual to see such a person here in Matlock. Even though this lady was a 'Chink', as we impolitely called her race, I was drawn to her. What was it that attracted me? No, she did not have tiny feet, as we had been told.

She was exquisite. Her clothing was simple, yet elegant, and her demeanour suggested that she was very sure of herself. Kindness flowed from her as she interacted with the child, who was also responding with the same assurance. She epitomised for me, all that I had been taught and believed that a lady should be. I had wanted to visit her country for years now, I realised but China had been off limits to the West for years. President Nixon had finally opened the doors, and here was an opportunity to go. I'm not going to let it pass, I thought and, for the first time in my married life, I took a stand and said,

'I'm going to China, with or without you, but I hope you will come.'

It worked and, in April 1983, after our visit to Cannes, we were on our way. We were sitting in Seattle Airport awaiting our flight to be called.

'Look,' said the man next to me, 'Mount Ranier, on the horizon, in all its splendour. Our lucky day,' he said.

Perhaps a good omen for our trip, I thought. We were aboard the plane and on our way to Kyoto Airport in Japan. It was a long, long flight. We crossed the International Dateline and 'today' became 'tomorrow'! As we entered the airport, we saw another group of Americans. This was the Symphony Orchestra from Fort Worth, Texas. They were to tour China for three weeks. As we tried to get our bearings there was a great to do. The orchestra members were to be sent home. They could not enter China. One of the Chinese table tennis players currently competing in the USA had defected. The orchestra were to be punished, but what about us? We were all right. We were scientific, whatever that means, whereas music was not. We sadly said goodbye to our countrymen and boarded one of two very small planes. All this planing and deplaning was because of our political problems with Korea, who would not allow us to fly in their airspace. So south we went, turning west after we have left the land mass behind us, then retraced those miles north to reach Beijing, flying in Chinese airspace. Our arrival there was scary.

The airport was huge but there was not a plane in sight, not even one parked. We were greeted by armed soldiers with fixed bayonets. Our passports were taken and kept and we were forcibly pushed to board a rickety bus and taken to our hotel. Where was the rest of our group? we wondered. We were told that their plane had developed engine trouble and had to put down in Shanghai, but they were on their way to join us. We all gave great sighs of relief when they joined us a few hours later. We applauded heartily when our countrymen from Texas appeared in the lobby the next day.

'What a trip,' said Hank. 'Didn't I tell you that it would be awful in this primitive country?'

Well, I had to agree. We'd had our fill of excitement and hoped things would go a bit more smoothly. This beginning did not look well for our trip to come. However, it was all I wanted it to be, culture, sightseeing, food and interaction with the people. We were one of the first Western tourist groups to visit China after it opened up. The populace gazed at us in amazement. Everything about us was different, but the one feature that stood out was our physical fairness. Wherever we were, and whenever they could, they reached out to touch us. We were intrigued by the small feet of the women and were surprised to see how few these were. Binding was no longer allowed. It was the children who fascinated me. Their interest was enormous, but was always displayed with respect and courtesy. Verbal communication was impossible, but we were amazed at how much could be conveyed by body and facial language. Our journey started in Beijing and we slowly made our way south to Hong Kong and our flight home.

Beijing was an attractive city, a mixture of old and new. There were people everywhere, with scarcely an inch between them. All the men were attired in the blue Mao jacket. It was an effort to get anywhere on foot and I was glad that we were not allowed to wander on our own. We were heavily guarded, not by the police but by our guides. One misguided couple knowingly strayed into forbidden territory, a hotel reserved for the local élite.

'Why should we not see what we want?' they asked.

'When in Rome, we do as Rome does,' they were told.

Our guide was severely censured and sent somewhere equivalent to Siberia, and no apology on our part could change the decision. Later, we learned that our companions' straying had resulted in demotion for the guide, even though he had had no idea of their plans and thus no way to stop them. We also learned that these guides' jobs were avidly sought after, for they offered an experience that few Chinese could avail themselves of, travel and most of all good food, for the authorities, in their efforts to encourage tourism, tended to cater to the American palate.

No one else in this great land mass ate as we did, neither the quantity nor the variety that we consumed. Indeed, we watched construction workers down a bowl of rice for lunch with three small leaves of lemon grass as a treat. Meat was a great luxury, as also was fish. We were expected to use chopsticks at mealtimes but I had brought my own fork and spoon, much to the envy of the other women. So imagine my distress when I could not find my utensils after forgetting to take them with me. Later they were rescued, for one thoughtful waiter had secreted them in a safe place. When I offered him a very small tip for his thoughtfulness, he shyly shook his head and refused. Actually the cuisine was very poor and nowhere near as good as American Chinese cuisine. We liked the beer and drank it at every opportunity, for, as in all foreign countries, we were advised not to drink the water.

Opposite our Beijing hotel was an empty block of flats. They were not inhabited, we were told, because the Russian builders could not get water to the higher storeys. In inhabited apartments we saw balconies used for all kinds of storage, furniture, bathtubs and firewood. Modern China was indeed, by our standards, poor in every way. Hygiene and sanitation left much to be desired. Our hotel had passable standards for both but, outside, it was all very primitive. Even in the better restaurants, toilets were mere holes in the floor. Squatting was the only way. In one restaurant, I entered the girls' room to see a group of my colleagues standing behind closed doors with their heads and shoulders exposed. Just like fillies in their stalls and all because we were so much taller than the average Oriental woman.

As we continued our journey, it became more and more obvious where a woman's place was. We hardly ever saw one outside. In one of the sweatshops they were sitting, cheek by jowl, stitching away for twelve straight hours. Grandmothers were the primary carers for the children and, just occasionally, we would see one pushing a wicker pram along the street.

A visit to one of the communes was revealing too. The one roomed houses had a curtain to be drawn at night for minimal privacy. There was an outdoor kitchen and a hole in the yard for the outhouse. There were no gadgets or appliances and few houses had any form of plumbing. Yet, this was within Beijing's city limits.

However deficient their way of life, nevertheless the cultural relics were overwhelmingly beautiful, both architecturally and culturally. There was splendour, splendour and more splendour. We walked along the Great Wall and were amazed at the number of men who expectorated in front of us. Were they telling us something, like Yankee go home? We were entertained to dinner in the Great Hall in Tianemen Square. We strolled through the Forbidden City and the Imperial and Summer Palaces. We loved the zoo and its pandas. I enjoyed watching the children, as they responded and reacted to the animals. I bought a cushion at the zoo which I needle pointed at my leisure. The panda on it still looks alive and real.

Our visit to Kindergarten Number One was a treat. I was entranced by these children. They were friendly, respectful, well behaved and controlled and very self-assured. Several gave little performances for us. They sang and danced and they were perfect. One child spontaneously offered me his drawing of the panda which he had just finished and it is still here amongst my souvenirs. We visited an adult psychiatric hospital and watched schizophrenics being treated with acupuncture. We visited the Children's Hospital. The wards were much like they had been in the West one hundred years ago, stark, cold and isolating. We saw few staff members and I don't know why. Acupuncture was very much in evidence. I was surprised to see two mothers with their children and wondered if this was to let us know that they were absorbing all the recent knowledge. Despite the primitive conditions, I felt very drawn to the people. They were friendly, respectful towards each other, self-controlled, family oriented and seemed highly motivated towards work and eager to do a good job. It was just like the world that I grew up in. I wondered what had changed humanity? Did technology help us to degenerate from a civil society?

We were scheduled to fly to our next destination late afternoon one Sunday. Our guide suggested that we should walk down the main street to the department store. What a throng of people there was. People, people, and more people were all around us. Was it really Sunday? Yes, it was and this was the main shopping day there, for everyone worked six days a week. Despite the hordes, business was sluggish. The street vendors, in spite of their cries and come-ons, were selling little.

The department store loomed up ahead. It was a solid brick modern building, with large revolving doors and large windows displaying all kinds of merchandise. It was very Western we thought. It took us a long time to get inside, for those doors revolved slowly – oh so slowly – and when we did get inside; wow! I could barely breathe, let alone move. Most people were heading for the escalator, a new addition to the store, we were told later. So we moved with the crowd. The escalator was a solid wall of people. Again, we were jammed against another human being. If this is togetherness, I don't want it, I thought. As we alighted from the escalator the crowd began to thin, as others hurried off in various directions. Even so, it became impossible to see much of the goods for sale. Business here was not brisk and I saw only one customer pick up a small package as he again merged with the crowd.

We arrived back at our hotel to learn that the flight had been cancelled. No reason had been given. We were now to travel by train. I was glad, for now we would interact with the natives and see more of the countryside. One couple believed that we were being cheated and insisted on being taken to the airport, as our schedule said. They were going to fly no matter what. Well, they were taken to the airport, as requested but, after we had been travelling in the train for some time, we stopped at a very small station and guess who got on. Yes! Our demanding couple. They had waited and waited and were finally convinced that there was no plane and the cab driver brought them to join the group. Who lost face in this predicament? The Orientals had played along with those unreasonable and incompatible Westerners.

Another incident amused us, too. We were all settled on the train and, just before we were to leave, an hotel employee rushed in requesting to talk to one of our group. He had found a ballpoint pen in the trash can. Did the owner really want to throw it away? The owner took it back, just so that that employee could save face, something that is very important here in the East.

Our next stop was Chang Sha in Hunan Province. Here, we were greeted by the Medical School staff. We were given a tour of the departments, and these were much as in Beijing. That evening, we were entertained at a banquet by the Professor of Paediatrics. Our menu escapes me now and the souvenir, that I still have, was written in Chinese.

We visited a primary school. It was very much like the kindergarten in Beijing. The children were older and many of them were learning to play musical instruments. Some performed for us and we were impressed by their competence. When we toured the building, we were surprised to see a group of six boys sitting in a line having their hair cut by older peers, all under the supervision of an adult.

We continued on our way to Canton. When we arrived at the hotel, we were informed that our reservations had been cancelled and given to a Chinese delegation. We were taken out into the countryside and housed in a fairly modern hotel amidst the rice paddies, lychee groves and where the water buffalo roamed with no respect for traffic or people. Not a smidgen of arable land was wasted and even along the railway embankments the soil was tilled and cultivated to the edges. When we arrived at the station in Canton, we were greeted by the orchestral group from Texas. They were happy with their tour, but were looking forward to getting back home. Our train carried us safely to Hong Kong through agricultural landscapes, all very well tended, all very soporific and there was never a tractor in sight, only the water buffaloes plodding behind ploughs, steered by plodding humans of various ages. That is the way that I always think of China after all these years. I wonder if modern civilisation has touched this vast land mass and if it has, has it changed the tempo and life style of its people?

Hong Kong was a bustling city with bustling people and many touches of Westernisation. We were booked into the Sheraton Hotel and felt that home was not so far away. Lunch time arrived and we all hurried to the coffee shop. They were expecting us and had good old Yankee food to hand, hamburgers and French fries, what else? What a good meal it was, even if it was not my favourite one. We all recognised that we had had more than our fill of rice and the Chinese cuisine. That night, we went to the dining room and enjoyed Western cooking again and also the ambience that accompanies a night out on the town, soft dulcet music and waiters running hither and thither. We saw all the sights of Hong Kong. For me, the most exciting part was riding, and then climbing, to the top of the mountain and drinking in the unbelievable and indescribable view. Best of all, I called Esther. The sound of her voice and home was just what I needed. It had been a wonderful trip, exotic, enlightening, instructional and with many memorable events and happenings, but I was weary and ready for my own bed. There's no place like home! I thought. The leopard never changes his spots. I liked my Western life and I was not anxious to change it.

On the long flight home, I wondered why the Chinese nation allowed itself to exist in such primitive conditions, whilst the rest of the world extended and over extended itself with materialism. Did the Chinese know what was happening in the outside world? I don't think so. Communication and the means for it were minimal. We saw few radios and not one television until we reached Hong Kong. Again I heard Mother's voice saying, 'One half the of world doesn't know how the other half lives.' It was true, true, true. I only knew that I didn't want to change my life style. Back home, our first challenge was to overcome the jet lag of twelve hours. The first day that I was back in the office, my secretary found me asleep at my desk at noon, midnight my time. She wakened me gently and I survived the afternoon challenges. Life just went on.

One More Massive Mission

While I was developing the school programme, Hank was also involved in a big venture. Shortly after we were married, the Professor of Paediatrics suggested that Hank send one of his Fellows to Atlantic City to be the Director of the Children's Seashore House. This was a programme for chronically ill children which had been established in the early 1900s to restore and care for city children suffering from chlorosis. This was an anaemic-like illness which responded only to fresh uncontaminated air.

'Wouldn't you like to do that?' I asked. 'It seems like an added extension of what you were doing in psychological paediatrics.'

After thinking it over, Hank agreed. He arranged to spend two days each week in Atlantic City and as the schedule evolved he chose to be there on Fridays and Mondays. As the weeks passed, we decided to find a small apartment there. We all liked the ocean and the beach and if we spent weekends by the briny, life would be easier for Hank. We found just what we wanted, next door to the hospital in the Warrick Apartments. On the seventh floor – a joke that we overused – we were safe, for the firemen's ladder would reach as far as the seventh floor, but no further. We all looked forward to Friday afternoons and our weekends by the ocean. Even winter seemed warmer there, but what hectic afternoons those Fridays turned into. Riding first, then hitting the AC Throughway. Well, we were young and energetic and full of life. We enjoyed this lifestyle for many years.

It ended when the Board of Governors decided to move the programme to Philadelphia and build a modern facility adjacent to the new Children's Hospital on the grounds of the old Philadelphia General Hospital. Well, that was one good result of casinos. For as these took over Atlantic City, it became more and more difficult to get staff and less and less therapeutic for the patients. It was a mammoth task and, as each stage was achieved, Hank and I had our own private celebration. At the grand opening, we dined at the same table as HRH Princess Margaret. Did I have to come all the way to the USA for this? I thought.

We lost our second home and missed it. Then one day, at lunch and just by chance, one of Hank's colleagues was talking of property on the Eastern Shore of Maryland. Hank's attention was grabbed and we were soon on our way to visit a realtor – Winfield Trice – in Hurlock. We had no idea what we wanted, but Winfield made us much more certain after grilling us for one hour. He introduced us to the Neck District of Cambridge and on a cold, wet and miserable day in January 1983 he showed us around an old waterfront farmhouse on Ross Neck Road. As soon as I saw it, I knew that it was for us. Hank was more reticent.

'That's it,' I said.

'We can't buy it just like that,' was the reply, but we did return the following week and made an offer. The owners – two brothers – were impossible. They did not agree about anything and, in March when we were in England, we said nothing about our plans. Why stir up excitement if it wasn't to be ours? we thought. On our return, they had finally agreed to our offer and terms and Littleworth Farm became ours. We had barely moved in when Sis and Eric arrived in the USA. They were our first guests. Even with the makeshift accommodation, they could see what I liked and agreed with me that it was a little piece of England transplanted on the wrong side of the briny. As the years have passed, we have spent many happy times mostly with family and friends and, at times, I must confess that I have felt like a motel manager, but every minute has been well worthwhile. So our life went on.

The Empty Nest

An empty nest had, finally, arrived, slowly but surely. As I entered from the garage, there was a quiet eeriness about the house, even on Thursdays despite Lessie, our maid, being there prior to my return from the office. Wait, there he was, Ollie, my best friend, alert and ready to jump whether it was friend or foe. It was me. He jumped down from his cosy couch, wagging his tail with his eyes aglow, pushing himself close, closer, until he was nuzzling me with his nose. There was no roughness. He quietly and gently begged with his eyes to be stroked. After our greeting, he watched and followed me, for this was his dinner time and, once he had eaten, it was his walking time. He looked forward to this and he became skittish and excited as I reached for his leash. Off we went, he pulling and leading the way. For he, just like me, had his preferences. We met some of the neighbours, either returning from their daily chores or walking their dogs. We stopped and chattered to some and bid others, 'good day'. Most recognised Ollie, as well as his mistress.

Then we went back home. What should we have for dinner? I thought. I set about preparing it and all would be ready when

Hank was ready to eat, but there was lots of time before then. I was home much earlier than he was. I settled on the couch with my latest book. Ollie settled comfortably beside me, content to be where he was. He didn't sleep or snooze and, at times, he gave me a little nudge just to let me know that he was there and to get a little attention, a soft word, a pat and a stroke. Time flew by and, before I knew it, the garage door groaned as it rose, signalling the master's arrival. Down went the book, up jumped Ollie and we moved into the kitchen to welcome him home with our usual kiss and Ollie's usual nudging. He settled in his favourite chair with the mail, and I set out our 'Happy Hour', on the porch in summer, or by the glowing wood stove in winter. Dinner went into the oven. Later, it waited, for the microwave fixed it quickly.

This was the happiest time of my day. We were together and we could share our day with concern or fun. Ollie shared it too, looking from one to the other as each one spoke. Then it was time to eat and on went the television and we dined to the accompaniment of Learer and Lerner. They held the stage and we listened critically to their news. Once we had finished eating and the dishes were out of the way, we settled down for the evening. Was there anything worth watching on television? we thought. Sometimes there was and we watched together. Sometimes there wasn't and I retreated with my book. He retreated into his paper. Sometimes there was something for him and again my book became my solace and my saviour. Despite our efforts to accept our situation we were both lonely. We were both aware of this and we both hated it. It seemed so lifeless, I said.

'Then let's get some life into our evenings,' he replied.

How? We had activity, for we continued to enjoy the opera, the orchestra, our favourite restaurants, our friends and the social life with them. As the weeks passed we both sank deeper into our professional lives and involvements. We seemed to be drawing apart. Perhaps we were not enjoying each other? Life offered us no real challenge in any area. Then, once again, life found a solution, for events brought our waterfront farm into our lives. Suddenly we were busy, busier and busier. Littleworth Farm filled our need for something to care for. It gave focus and purpose to our lives again, and care for that farm we did. Each Friday morning, I packed, and each Friday afternoon after work we set off for the Eastern Shore. Our friends, Sally, Doe and Joe, joined us on most weekends and, with their help, we began to restore the 1839 structure to a semblance of its original self. One of our friends was an expert on the architecture of that period and both male friends were excellent carpenters. Both my female friends were good painters and one was an excellent cook. After several weeks of teamwork, we called ourselves 'The Golden Wonders'. For none of us had expected to be involved with a project such as we had undertaken at Littleworth Farm. Inside and outside, the work went on.

When we had the farm in shape, several years later, I shipped over the furniture from England that Mother had left to me. It was just right. Mother had hoped that we would retire in England, thus the furniture and, although she would have been disappointed that we had not returned home, she would have been pleased with our little farm and how well the furniture fitted. Well, even though I missed returning to my homeland, I now felt as though my homeland had come to me, for Littleworth Farm truly felt like home. All the furniture had been in my home as I was growing up, some had even been in my own room. Now all those memories would be part of my daily living, and so, in 1986, three years after we had acquired it, Littleworth Farm became my piece of transplanted homeland – England – and we spent every weekend and some weeks there for nine months of each year. I wondered if those early settlers had had similar thoughts and feelings. Well, it was no matter. Once again some extraneous force had solved our problem and kept us on the right track. So life went on!

The Santa Fe Years: More Sorrow and Sadness

The phone rang. It was Jim from Santa Fe. He sounded quite upset and something must be wrong for he never called just to chat. He left that to his wife. Yes, he did have some upsetting news. Mary had been hospitalised following her second miscarriage. She was in no danger, but she was very upset. She had so wanted a second child and she had been extra happy when she had conceived, but now, a second miscarriage. As usual, she blamed herself, even though no physical or medical reason had been discovered. Worst of all, she had been told that she must not conceive again. All hope had been taken away. Eddy would be an only child, which was something that she did not want for him.

I flew out when she returned home and she was very down. How could I help her? She was only a little weak physically and preferred to run her house and care for Eddy. It kept her connected and took her mind off her problem. When we were alone she wanted to talk, which was something new in our relationship. I was there for her and so I listened. She shared some of her earlier unhappiness with her own problem, some of the happiness and satisfactions of motherhood and how she would never feel these again. She talked of her unhappiness and her poor efforts to care for her own mother during the latter's psychotic episodes, and how responsible she felt for her brother's care, at least in feeding and sleeping, even though she was only three years his senior. She spoke of her anger and resentment when I came into the family. Her biggest worry was her fear that she may be diabetic. She had recently experienced some trouble with her eyes, but she had not consulted her physician. I just felt that she knew this was her problem and that she was delaying its confirmation, but we must get this question answered, especially as her natural mother had suffered from this illness and died alone in a diabetic coma.

So, an appointment was made and the tests were performed. Yes, there it was, the diagnostic blood sugar pattern confirming the disease. Yes, this could be the cause for those miscarriages. Treatment was not too difficult. She was readily stabilised on insulin and she could control her diet. She quickly became competent in caring for herself, blood testing, diet control and medication. This afforded her some solace, but it only intensified her disappointment and frustration. The family settled down. Mary returned to her regular life and I returned home.

Another year passed and she and Eddy came east to visit us. The diabetes continued to be well controlled and her health and life went on as usual, but she still wanted another child and she was actively exploring adoption, even though Jim was averse to this. She was verbally encouraged by one of her cousins who had recently adopted twins. She openly discussed the pros and cons with us and we expressed our own feelings and beliefs on the subject. I found lots of research articles on the pros and cons and some on the outcome of adoptive efforts.

Months later, the phone rang and it was Mary. She and Jim had finally hashed the problem over and they were going to find a baby to belong to them. They had registered with an agency in the east – Virginia, I think – but this was no easy matter. Available infants were few and far between, but they were going to try. They were fully supported by all Jim's family and their Quaker friends, and news from the cousin and her efforts was very encouraging. Still, I remained sceptical. Another year passed. Eddy was now six and Mary's longing for another infant had increased, as he became more and more independent.

Then, it happened. An infant born on 26 April was in need of a home. They agreed to bring him into the family. He was Afro-American and this was a southern family. There was a great to do, but they were adamant and he arrived at their home in Santa Fe when he was just three weeks old. He was an attractive, healthy, bouncing boy. He settled down in the family quickly. Mary felt quite confident in caring for him and he was accepted by Jim and Eddy. It was hard for Eddy, who had been the centre of attention of both parents, but he struggled with having to share his parents.

'Anyway, I'm bigger than Joey, and now I'm like my friends, I've got a brother,' he said. So, life went on.

Retirement

Yes, life went on. The children were settled or settling into their own lives. We were settled comfortably into our two homes. Our careers were flourishing and we had time on our hands. Most of all, we had time for each other, something we had never had before. We only had ourselves to consider now.

It was 1987 and I was eligible to retire. But this was the last thing that I wanted to do. I was healthy, fit, vigorous, and I loved life. Most of all, I loved my job, a job truly created by me. For, over the years, I had introduced and welded child psychiatry with education and, it had, through special education, been a success. Now the politicians were interfering with our programme, not only with the funding but with the processes and procedures which had been worked out from our clinical experience, and the programme was falling short. I did all that I could to fight this, both within the educational system and within the political system, but to no avail. I could not stand by and watch that good programme be destroyed.

Sadly, I decided to retire. After all, a voice within me said, 'You are well known within the community and you know most of the senior child psychiatrists. There should be another job somewhere.' So after a very touching retirement party, I said farewell to my friends and colleagues of many years. I had held that job for twenty-four years. I hated retirement. I had no place to go to and no purpose to life. One purposeless day followed after another. If there was nothing to get up for, I thought, why get up? I felt an awful sense of nothingness – just like when I faced that empty nest. I consoled myself by seeking out all the household chores that had been neglected. New drapes were needed here, perhaps, new cushion covers there. Perhaps... no, I don't think so. A coat of paint on that door, well, we'll see. What about the garden? I'll tell Bill to lop the bushes and mend the fence, I thought.

Our usual question on meeting at the end of the day, 'How

was your day?' gradually faded, for Hank knew what I was going to reply.

Then one day he said, 'Let's take a break. Let's go and see Chuck in Florence and see how he is making out.'

What a great idea, I thought. So we set our lives in order and booked our passage to Rome!

Chuck and Firenzi

Chuck was the son of Alice and Charles, Hank's older brother. I first met him at our wedding. At that time, he was a senior at Nutria High School in Winnetka, Illinois, and he was beginning to look at colleges in the eastern USA. He finally elected to attend Haverford College in Bryn Mawr, very close to our neighbourhood. Thus we got to know him very well, for he became a member of our family, and I, his surrogate mother. He spent many hours with us and he and Hank had mutual interests in art. After graduating from Haverford, he moved to Yale. We missed him, of course, but we kept in touch, even when he moved to Europe and finally settled in Florence. We attended his wedding in Marblehead, Massachusetts, and continued to hear about him through his parents. His life was typical of that of most artists, with ups and downs, but his parents stood firmly behind him in his ventures and he slowly made headway. His first child had been born two years ago, and we were anxious to meet this new member of the clan. So our trip to Italy was planned.

My friend Sally was to fly with us to Rome, where she would meet up with her son, a lawyer on a business trip to Rome, Milan and Pisa. Then my sister, Sis would meet us in Florence, where we would also be joined for a few days by my friend, Marga, who would drive down from Bertchesgarden with a friend and be with us for a few days. Thus we would catch up with some very special people in my life and share some happy times and adventures together. It all worked out as planned and with some extra excitement to give the trip a little spice. Our flight from Philadelphia landed in Roma. What a commotion we found at the airport.

Italy had a reputation at that time for its sudden and unexpected strikes. Here we were, in the midst of one of them. There was a general transportation strike. Everyone had to use a private vehicle or taxi cab to move around the city. Our first task was to locate a cab. It was not at all easy. We pushed and were pushed. Finally we achieved success. We piled into the first cab available and directed the driver to take us to the Elite Hotel. He nodded his head, giggled incessantly and repeated constantly, 'Ito, Ito, Ito.' We did not know what he was saying but thought that it was related to the traffic. It was something to behold, bumper to bumper for as far as we could see and in every lane. We swayed to the constant stopping and starting for over an hour. Then he took a sharp turn to the left, where there was no other car, put his foot down and, lo and behold, he was waving his hands in great delight. We were outside the Hilton Hotel. We looked perplexed and confused. We tried to tell him the name of our hotel, but more confusion followed. We wrote down the hotel's name. 'Ah,' he said with relief, but now, we were back into the sea of traffic again. We were across the city from our destination. After another hour of swaying, another swerve, this time to the right, there it was, our hotel! We couldn't wait to get out of the cab. What a welcome to such an ancient, yet modern, European capital.

The strike continued for the rest of our stay in Rome, but we had a little more control over our movements as we got to know our way around. Sally's son, Preston, was a great help for he spent quite some time each year in the city. After a short rest, we felt up to exploring on shank's pony. There was no more riding that day. I don't recall all the places that we visited, nor in what order we visited them, but I do remember that the Spanish Steps were within walking distance from the hotel, and so they were easily available to us. I relived that afternoon, looking at the photograph, I remember that it was a lovely sunny afternoon. Hordes of people were climbing up and down the steps. Then we admired a flower stall just at the bottom of the steps with the most magnificent display of temperate and tropical flowers, much as one sees in New York, London or Paris. The view from the top of the steps made up for the great energy needed to reach the top.

After a delicious dinner, Italian cuisine of course and nothing like the American apology, and a good night's sleep, we were raring to cover more territory the next day. The Coliseum was awe inspiring. As a British subject I was used to old buildings and old cities, but I had not seen anything like this. How could a building exposed to wind and weather have withstood the ravages of time so well? I thought. We could visualise this arena filled with throngs of cheering crowds and imagine the jostling as they came and went. The places that I liked the most were the piazzas. Here in those small secluded enclaves, with their small stores, ristorantes and gelateria, one could be seated comfortably and satiate one's craving for genuine Italian cuisine and water ices and, at the same time, watch the people. We soon learned how to pick out the natives from the tourists. The former always seemed so directed and earnest, the latter relaxed and overwhelmed. For the ambience of those ancient buildings was awe inspiring and breathtaking. We frequented the Piazza Navona because of its wonderful fare, but the most beautiful piazza for me was the Piazza Del Populo, with its Church of Saint Mary and the Caravaggio paintings. I could have stayed there all day. In that dignified silence and the themes of the paintings, life's purpose became more certain and clearer.

Then there was Saint Peter's Square. We attended a papal audience, all the while hanging on to our pocket books and wallets – as recommended by those in the know – lest they become fodder for the gypsy gamins whose sole purpose was to pick the pocket of the unwary, a task that they were well versed in and at which they excelled. We wandered through Saint Peter's Church and the Sistine Chapel, drinking in Leonardo's masterpieces, as well as the Pieta. Then we went to the Trevi Fountain into which we dropped our coins singing, 'Five Coins In the Fountain' just as many others had done ahead of us. Then, on the way back to the hotel, our route took us by a quite unexpected building, a pyramid. Yes, it was authentic, but I cannot recall the details of its origin all these years later.

One afternoon, we strayed far from the hotel. We were tired and needed a cab to take us back. What a to do it was to get one. Finally, as we were standing amidst swirling traffic, one kind cabbie saw our distress and took his life into his hands to reach us on the other side of the sea of cars. No hotel bed had ever felt so good as mine after so intense a day. Then, we set off to Florence – Firenzi – and our visit with Chuck and his family. We boarded our train, which took us through some of the most beautiful country in Italy. Waiting at our hotel, in the Piazza Santa Maria Novello, was my sister and we were later joined by Marga and her friend who had driven down from Bertchesgarden. There was so much excitement, so much catching up to do. That evening, we had a reunion dinner at the local ristorante – Il Profito – and agreed to meet for breakfast and plan our programme for the next few days. We called Chuck to see how we could fit into his busy teaching schedule. Chuck and Isobelle were home. They agreed to join us for dinner that evening. We met at Ristorante Il Profito and had a little celebratory dinner, which everyone enjoyed. Then they walked us back to the hotel and outlined our sightseeing programme.

Florence was a relatively small city and most of the tourist attractions were within walking distance. The city's ambience enfolded us and no matter where we looked there was no invasion of the ancient by the modern. Our first attraction was the Church of Santa Maria Novello, within the same piazza as our hotel. Its imposing façade was welcoming and we particularly liked its cloisters. We also liked the Church of San Croce, again with its imposing façade, this time in marble, and the tombs of Michelangelo, Galileo, Rossini and Dante. The Palazzo Vecchio was the most imposing and majestic building in Florence. It was solid, definite and looked as though it would withstand any assault or onslaught. It had been standing since the late thirteenth century and showed no noticeable evidence of wear and tear. This Palazzo dominated the Piazza Della Signoria, and we soon discovered our favourite eatery, the Ristorante Il Latino in that most famous and beautiful square. It was there in that piazza, over the centuries, that the great political and historical events of the city took place. The square became the symbol of the internal struggles in Florence, the establishment of its international prestige and power, and the civilisation and culture which it had given to the world.

The Pitti Palace, considered the most monumental building in Florence, was started in the middle of the fifteenth century by Brunelleschi for Luca Pitti, a very rich merchant and rival of the Medici family. He wanted a residence larger than any built in

Florence and with windows larger than the entrance door of the Medici Palace in Via Larga. Well, even then, pride went before a fall and, in 1465, the Pitti family was financially ruined. The buildings were rescued by various Florentine families and, finally, the Medici's and their successors, the Lorraines, rescued it and it became the royal palace of the Savoy dynasty during the period when Florence was capital of Italy. Each room was magnificent in its own way, with gilded frescos and ceilings and walls laden so heavily with Renaissance paintings that one's eye was constantly distracted from one masterpiece to another.

It was just the same, in the Uffizi Gallery. This imposing square and building were originally built by Vasari in 1560 to house the government administration offices. It, too, was overwhelming and I could only take in a little at a time. So I returned on three or four occasions, and I began to realise what they meant by tourist flu. The weather was perfect and, when satiated, I would repair to one of the open air cafés and relax with a cup of tea before the nausea occurred, and recoup my strength.

The Bobolo Gardens was another must. Here the magnificent statuary was tastefully scattered throughout and the impact was far less intent, less overwhelming and easier to assimilate. The River Arno flowed through Florence and the vistas of the river and the city was magnificent. It was enhanced by the numerous bridges which spanned the water. The most famous of these bridges was the Ponte Vecchio. It is the oldest bridge in Florence and has been in existence since AD 972. The original wooden bridge was destroyed by floods and it was reconstructed in stone in 1345, with the shops alongside, just as they are today. These were originally rented to butchers but, at the wish of Cosimo the First, they were reassigned to gold and silversmiths and it has continued much this way. High up on the left side of the bridge, ran the Vasari Corridor connecting the Uffizi Gallery with the Pitti Palace.

Despite all the elegance and beauty of Florence, the most memorable vistas for me were of the city from the Piazza Michelangelo, the most magnificent view of the River Arno dividing the city, the bridges spanning the river and the hills surrounding the city. It was a sight that could not be missed. The

Piazza itself was one of the most attractive, with its statue to Michelangelo in the centre. Another panoramic view that must not be missed was that seen from Fiesole. It was an exciting trip, for the ride into the mountains offered spectacular scenery, the little village had a charm of its own and then below lay Florence in all its glory.

Well, what a breathtaking experience it had been! We were sated with knowledge of the Renaissance era. To celebrate our tourist efforts, we had dinner at our favourite ristorante. There was a sadness in the air as we gathered, for this was to be a farewell meal as well as a celebration. We said goodbye to Sally and Preston who were off to Milano and Pisa. We said goodbye to Marga and her friend, as they started to wend their way back to Bertchesgarden. Tomorrow, we would be just a threesome – Hank, Sis and me. On the eve of departure day, the phone rang. It was Marga. She had forgotten to pick up her passport from the hotel office. She asked if I would be good enough to take it to the German Embassy. They would make sure that it was returned to its rightful owner. All went as predicted. She called the next day. It was back with its owner again.

We were joined by Chuck, who took us to his apartment. It was located in one of the older palaccios in the city. It was a stone building with a classical Florentine façade. We started to climb, up, up, up – all eighty-four steps – all very well worn and thus very easy to take in our stride. The door was opened by Isobelle, his French wife, whom we had met at their wedding three years ago. We were introduced to her daughter, Sara, who had grown since we last met. She was a pretty eight or nine year old now and very competent socially. Then, the pièce de résistance, their daughter Charlotte, a lively outgoing two year old.

We were impressed by the comfort and convenience of the apartment, which had been renovated carefully from the old building, maintaining the feel of age and permanence. It was cosily furnished in the European style and the walls displayed several of Chuck's artistic creations. One, 'The Blind Man', caught the eye. It was so demanding of attention that I and others were continually drawn to it during dinner. The meal was ready and waiting and we were invited to be seated at the table, We drank a toast to ourselves and to each other and then wallowed in the excellent cuisine – Italian with just a hint of Francaise.

'The Blind Man' continued to intrude in our socialising. He intrigued us and no wonder, for this canvas won a prize for Chuck and gave him entrance into the artistic world in Florence. As a result, he had started a small art school for English and American students and his British name had opened many doors for him and his school.

He promised to show us his studio the next day and, when we visited it, there were several students at their easels. Their paintings were in various states and stages of development. Chuck believed that his own forté lay in portraiture and we could see from his paintings that this seemed to be so. He was beginning to expand his skills and move into still life and landscapes. I was enamoured of one of the latter painted in the Tuscan Hills and, much later on, I became the proud possessor of this canvas.

We kept in touch with Chuck over the years, both personally and through his parents. Many years later, we were able to convince the Board of Governors at the Seashore House that he should be selected to Hank's portrait in recognition of the work that he had done in establishing the new building and programme. This, in turn, led to subsequent portraitures of other well known Philadelphia physicians. He came over during the summer semester and stayed with us whilst completing these. Whilst life had its ups and downs for all of us, I was hoping that he and Charlotte would visit us at Yuletide and we could catch up on all that had happened to all of us.

All Good Things Come to an End

We were back in the old US of A. It was good to be home. All had gone well without us around. The weekend was over and it was back to the daily round and common task. The euphoria of our trip faded. A solemness seemed to overcome us. We weren't quite so free as we had been. We both seemed more subdued. Was it true, or was it just my own way of getting back in harness? Were we happy? Again I thought so, but could I bear it if this was not so? Hank had never been openly affectionate, or expressive of his feelings and emotions. Whenever I tried to express happiness beyond just the verbal, with a look or touch, he always withdrew. If I tried to have a discussion about our interaction, I was immediately stopped, verbally, with some trite accusation or blame, or by his just removing himself from the scene. Talking about our problems was 'verboten'.

The topic and the problem were swept under the rug, and there they remained. So we went through the physical motions of existing and living. What had happened to those intimate moments of sharing, the quiet jokes together, the mystery of the beloved. As I had grown older, I had seen how Mother and Dad had had their brand of intimacy, the quiet voice, the gentle touch, the arched eyebrow! Where was this in my life? Had it ever been there? There had always been too many intrusions between us, but these were gone now. Could we not develop this aspect of our relationship, now that we had no one to intrude, or witness our overtly expressed feelings for each other? We had all the time in the world to test ourselves out, but no discussion was allowed.

Was this a stage in the game of life? I asked myself. Some of my friends were experiencing the same relationship problems in their lives. Wira's marriage had ended in divorce, leaving her shattered, disillusioned and alone. One by one, several of our colleagues announced pending separation and divorce. What was happening? Someone invented the term mid-life crisis and the media played this to the hilt. Did our generation need children to keep us together? Was it the newly liberated females who were at fault? Articles proclaiming trophy babies born to young women, the second wives of middle-aged men, almost encouraged this as a new Americanism. Were we caught up in this new social moral scene? Still, no discussion was allowed! Even after an unhappy weekend at the Waldorf, no discussion, or thought of planning around whatever it was, was allowed! So life went on in its not so merry way.

Then, we were suddenly again a threesome. Joe was included in every thing we did. He joined us at the opera, at the orchestra, at dinner and movies. Every Monday night after dinner, Hank went off to Joe's house and allegedly to his workshop, just for a bit of male company. This from a man whom, for years, I had tried to encourage to stop off at the Faculty Club for just that purpose, but all to no avail. Was this the way American life evolved? I thought. The literature did not suggest so, but this was modern America, the country that won World War Two and allowed its Veterans to do what they liked! Well we'd just live with it and see what evolved, I decided. So life went on.

So Life Goes On

The holidays came and went. Esther and her friend and Jim and his friend joined us for Thanksgiving. We enjoyed the usual routines, the parade in Philadelphia, lunch at Hymies and the usual festive fare at home for dinner. Then it was Christmas. As usual, the children with or without friends, as well as my sister, joined us for Christmas Eve and Christmas Day. The tree was, as usual, the centre of our festivities. Then off we went to Santa Fe and the other half of the family. Eddy was three that year and very much aware of Christmas and its goodies. Just to watch that small boy gave an added dimension to my life.

We came home again and a long cold winter faced us. How we counted the days to opening up the farm! One cold and snowy day, the phone rang.

'It's Rehana,' the voice said.

It was one of the child psychiatrists who had worked with me and was now the Director of the Adolescent Unit at Norristown State Hospital.

'How's it going? she asked.

I tried to put on a good front, but Rehana wasn't fooled. Hadn't she told me that I would hate retirement?

'I know that you were not happy, whiling away the time,' she said.

She had called to tell me that she needed another staff child psychiatrist, starting in March, and to see if I'd like to join her staff. She knew what I was going to say and we both were happy and satisfied. Manna from Heaven again. So began another interesting and different professional experience for me.

The Norristown Forensic Unit

On 1 March 1988, I returned to work and a focussed life again. It was another new beginning, new staff, new patients and a whole new world. I really knew nothing about the legal profession and the men in charge, but I must remember that I was a physician and think in those terms. I was both excited and wary. Would it be like working with the educators? Yes! I expected that it would, for people were people, no matter what their calling. Well, good luck, Patsy, I thought. Another new era was dawning.

The drive to the hospital was easy, and parking was plentiful. I found the right building after cruising around. It was a typical square brick building, somewhat isolated and off the beaten track. It was not very accessible to any major entrance to the grounds, which of course were limited by high cement walls topped with barbed wire due to someone's good thinking!

As usual, I was five minutes early. Dad's good training still held fast. But Rehana was there, ready and waiting. She greeted me and took me to my office. It had a nice familiar feeling, but needed a little touch here and there to make it feel like mine. That would come. We went to the wards, where work was in progress and she introduced me to the staff, medical and nursing.

There were two other physicians, Sid Altman, my peer, whom I had known for many years and a young fellow, Jim Feusner who had been through my programme in the public schools but had decided to specialise in forensic psychiatry, a new branch of psychiatry which was just developing. We were all invited to join the head nurse for coffee whilst she initiated me into the practices and procedures of the ward. Each physician had his own caseload of patients for whom he was responsible. If he was absent, as he frequently was due to attendance in court, then whoever was available was responsible for providing whatever was needed, medication, isolation, physical restraints, etc. Thus we got to know all the patients and they got to know us. Since we all had had similar training, this created little problem, but it was the head nurse who really kept us going, as she tactfully interacted with us. If we seemed perplexed or unclear what to do, or we did not know what was needed, she would quietly whisper the solution in our ear and we would gratefully follow her advice. Once again, I learned a lot from the nursing staff, who had had so much more experience than I had.

As I look back, I believe that this was the hardest job that I ever had. The patients were not really sick. They were deviant. They did not fit the human mould. Their ages ranged from fourteen to eighteen and all had committed one or more serious crimes such as arson, murder, or robbery. All had serious criminal consequences to face. I had to look at my own attitude toward this youth group. The hardest part for me was the total lack of remorse, expressed or displayed by those, yes, let's face it, young criminals. Theirs was a different but characteristic personality. They all showed a social unrelatedness, no empathy and an intense distrust of all other humans, peers and adults alike. They were aware of this, frequently expressed it and used it as a self-protective device, essential for self-survival.

Even though they knew right from wrong and admitted to the wrongness of their behaviour, they were not sorry for whatever they had done and tended to blame others for it. All responded impulsively without any thought or concern for the consequences to themselves or others. All denied remorse for damage or injury, resulting from their behaviour. Socialisation was inhibited and few expressed a wish for any close relationship with peer or adult. Our earlier research had suggested that this had occurred due to a lack of attachment in early life, which in turn resulted in developmental delay in the areas of interpersonal relationships and impulse control for the regulation of aggressive behaviour. These findings had been confirmed as recently as 1997, and long after our own conclusions.

How were we to help those youths? we asked ourselves. Earlier attempts had been quite unsuccessful. As I began to interact with the group, it struck me that they did not trust anyone, but each person handled this differently. Some just laughed in the other's face, some became belligerent, some withdrew, but, no matter, all demeaned the other person. What we needed to get to was the reason. This was impossible for, covered up, was intense rage, of which they were not aware. Whenever they were threatened, this came to the surface and they had no in-built mechanism to help to control their reactions. Therapy was really a waste of time, whether on an individual or group basis. Logic was always distorted, and reason was made fun of. We did resort to behaviour modification techniques in the hope that we could help to develop whatever assets each youth possessed, and some, particularly in the younger group, did begin to view the world and their place in it in a kindlier light.

All these youths were in the custody of the courts and this necessitated our working closely with judges, lawyers and probation officers on a monthly basis. Once all of the legal verbiage was over, the basic question for all of us was, 'What did those criminals need?' They were not really mentally ill. They were deviant. Their perceptions of life and the way they reacted to it was because of those perceptions, which had developed over the years as a result of their own experience with other humans. Our goal, it would seem, must be to help to change their distorted perceptions, help them develop more realistic ones, and learn to socialise appropriately, so that they could feel good about themselves and other human beings in whatever role they were interacting. It all sounded very logical, but how did one change the way that they felt and thought?

We started with the environment. Could we create a living milieu which would provide limits, boundaries, rules and regulations, geared to supporting growth in the self and with each other. The idea of residential placement was born. This was not to be a punitive environment, but a growth enhancing one, with supportive staff available as needed, with educators and technicians. The goal was to help each youth to develop himself personally and socially so that he could find and hold down a job for which he was trained. To qualify, each youth had to meet required standards and this was for us the hard part. Our behaviour modification gave us a start and, on the whole, our legal colleagues were supportive of our efforts.

We had just got everything in place when Sid became seriously ill and was no longer able to work. We struggled on with two of us trying to hold the fort. It was not very easy, for now we had to attend more and more court appearances. Then Jim was offered a job that he had wanted for some time. So, now, there was only me with a totally impossible job to do. Added to that was the fact that the state refused to hire anyone else, as it was now known that the Adolescent Unit was to move to another campus. It was more than I could cope with, and it was with great sorrow that I said goodbye to Rehana, who bore me no ill-will. A few days later, I found a letter awaiting me from one of the Mental Health Clinics in the city, asking if I could help them to develop a partial hospital programme and a crisis programme and would I consider meeting with them the next day. Well, what did I have to lose? At least I would not be bored and lonely again, and so my second retirement came and went.

The Community Council

I knew the building at 4900 Wyalusing Avenue in Philadelphia well, for it once housed the school for delinquent boys and I was frequently called over by the principal for consultations with staff and for student evaluations. Well, it was a little bit like returning home. I had lots of ambivalent feelings and thoughts running through my head. I was immediately shown into the director's office and after a pleasant half hour together, she called in Dr Roslin Smith, the chief adult psychiatrist. I had known Dr Smith when she was a student so, again, our interview went well. In essence, the agency needed to develop a children's programme and she needed a child psychiatrist to do it. This was to be a different programme – not just evaluating and diagnosing children for outpatient treatment. Now, we needed to develop a crisis unit, in which children at risk from self-harm and suicide could be seen and evaluated immediately and referred to appropriate programmes for treatment and, most of all, for self-protection during the crisis hours or days.

The other need for the agency was to develop, with the Board of Education, programmes for children who, because of their deviant thinking and behaviour, were seriously underachieving academically and who were not responding to the services that they received in the special education programmes within the regular schools. Well, that was the challenge. I did seem to have some of the right qualifications and experience to help me with this challenge and so I started.

In many ways, this was one of the most exciting and satisfying jobs that I ever held. I kept my relationships within the school system, since the partial hospital programmes were staffed by teachers whom I had known previously and were supervised by the district special education supervisor, another person whom I had known and helped to grow and develop into his present job. I was working with mental health staff who were anxious to make a success of this new concept. It was very gratifying for all of us to watch the students respond slowly to the staff's input and although the changes were very slow, at least the students were maintained in a school environment and continued to succeed academically. After two years in the programme most students had matured sufficiently, both socially and academically, to return to the special education programmes in a regular school environment.

One very special personal gain was that I became friendly with two very competent Indian women social workers who had recently emigrated to the USA. We socialised together at lunch times, and they introduced me to their culture and cuisine. They would bring home-made Indian dishes, often leftovers from supper the night before, and so I was given the opportunity to sample wonderful curries, which Mother had given me samples of as I grew up. Also chapati, a flat bread, which I had previously sampled at Dudley Road Hospital, rice dishes made with the special Basmati rice, and a wonderful potato and rice dish, this time with a flat rice unique to India, the name of which I did not know. This was the beginning of our staff weekly luncheon meetings, to which we all brought our individual and unique cuisines. Our director encouraged these gastronomic affairs as he, too, was a well known gourmet! These menus ranged from soul food to Italian and Chinese dishes. Nobody knew from week to week what would be offered by each of us. Yes! the way to a man's and a woman's heart was through the stomach and our gastronomic sessions certainly united us as people and professionals. I think that this was the friendliest and most co-operative group of professionals that I ever worked with.

We needed to co-operate with each other. For our work was at times very stressful, particularly in the crisis unit. The work here was hard, intense and disturbing. It consisted of making judgements from interviews with both patient and carers. Not much was conveyed by physical evaluations and even interviewing patients was not excessively revealing. Putting the information from both parties together gave the best sense of what was happening in the patient's life at that particular time and gave some indication of his level of vulnerability and need for protection against self-harm, in other words his need for hospitalisation.

The skill for me was not so much in the diagnosis of the patient, but in convincing the hospital admitting physician of the child's need for admission and protection. As we worked closely with the several hospital employees, we developed good and trusting relationships together and they soon realised that we only referred patients who were really in need of their services. Usually we had no problems but then a new physician arrived in town and he was very difficult to convince. He believed that we were only trying to pass the buck on to him. Then, one day, I saw a sixteen year old girl who had made recurrent attempts at suicide for which she had been hospitalised on many occasions. This was always an alerting message. Added to this, she told me in no uncertain terms that she was going to succeed and nobody was going to stop her. Well, after one hour's discussion over the phone, I finally wore him down. He agreed to accept her, but with poor grace. The next day, a call came from the medical examiner's office requesting my evaluation. Apparently, although admitted to the hospital, she had killed herself by hanging herself with her belt during the night. Well, sometimes one could win, but only by a hair. So another eight years passed.

During that time, many changes occurred in the health care services and HMOs took over. Job descriptions and funding were in a state of flux. Worst of all, the neighbourhood changed. It was now a high level drug area. Dealing and using intensified and we would arrive at the building around half past eight to find mattresses strewn around the parking lot and needles and vials scattered here and there. This was despite intense security. Then came a fatal day. We arrived at the building to find a dead body on the steps. For me this was the end, for, as an elderly white woman, I no longer felt safe traversing the area, even in the light. When the second body was found, despite intensified security, I knew that it was time for me to go, and so I retired for the third time!

Just after I had made this known, I found a letter awaiting me on my desk from Dr Williams PhD, a psychologist whom I had known and worked with in the clinic.

'I know that you are leaving the clinic. Come and help me out,' he wrote.

When I talked with him, he said that he had just received a big grant to evaluate the needs of adolescent criminals currently in the Juvenile Justice Department. They had only limited staff and facilities and did not know what to do, or how to help the ever-increasing influx of delinquent and criminal youth. How could I refuse? Here was just the opportunity that I wanted to do a retroactive study on a group that I had been able to predict would develop unless early interventive efforts were made through the schools.

Of course, nobody had listened. Now, perhaps, I would have the proof that they could understand. So, once more I moved into another office and the job began. Despite the unstable life that these youths had experienced, all had records of their developmental progress starting early in life. One thing stood out. All had experienced early childhood deprivation and all had shown antisocial behaviour early in their school experience. Yes, another paper to write – the finale to my work that started thirty years ago, that had flourished through my clinical practice and now could really be validated. The paper, *The Antecedents of Antisocial Personality – Suggestions for Early Intervention*, was submitted to the AACAP but was not accepted because it was at that time politically incorrect.

India, 1989

Life went on, but not very happily. Hank became more and more morose. He had not as yet retired and he constantly admitted that he had no wish to retire. He loved his work and it gave meaning to his life. A younger physician had been appointed to be the Director of the Seashore House, and Hank had been appointed to be the head of the department for peer reviews. Now, all staff members were regularly reviewed regarding their clinical performances. Hank did not mind this. He had known the staff for many years and they him, so no one was really threatened. It did begin to tell on him and, as the thought of finally having to retire loomed ominously on the horizon, he became more and more withdrawn, wrapped up in himself and preoccupied. Even his memory seemed to become impaired.

Finally, he arranged to see a psychiatrist and was diagnosed as depressed and medicated with the latest highly toxic anti-depressants. It was all to no avail. So he once again in his life entered a therapeutic relationship with the professor of psychiatry at one of the medical schools in the city. Nothing seemed to change for better or worse, but life settled into some kind of pattern, nothing like we had known before. There was no togetherness, no jokes, no fun. Everything seemed to be an effort. We moved further apart. Each of us did our own thing and I began to feel like a robot, responding as expected rather than as me. I needed a break. So I suggested that we get away from it all. A new milieu, perhaps would help and so, in November 1989, we joined a group from the Medical Society and flew from J.F. Kennedy Airport to Heathrow Airport and then on to New Delhi, India.

Because of my increasing socialisation with my Indian social worker friends, I was very curious to visit their country, not just to see the sights. Although I had always thought of the Taj Mahal in a romantic way, I wanted to see the populace as it lived and worked, to feel some of the ambience of the cities and countryside and learn a little of their history. New Delhi was an impressive city with big wide streets, magnificent government buildings, green parks and gardens. There was much hustle and bustle and, despite its modernity, fragments of an older and more primitive civilisation continued to force themselves on us. Rickshaws were everywhere and somehow seemed to me to emphasise the discrepancy between class and caste. How could one man sit calmly amid so much traffic whilst his brother, usually barefoot, pulled him along, like an oxen or a horse? Only I seemed upset.

The city was immaculate and very clean, thanks to the labouring of a squad of middle-aged men with besom brooms, and this despite the sacred cows wandering freely on all the highways leaving plasters of excrement wherever it would drop.

On one side street, we came across one sacred cow in labour. Everything had stopped and, without too much ado, the calf was born, attended to by its mother and slowly, together, they moved to the sidewalk, freeing the street for the traffic again. In such situations, the rickshaws were a blessing, since they could circumnavigate these domestic events.

Old Delhi was very old. The buildings were obviously ancient and of quite unique architecture. Hindu and Moslem temples loomed high into the sky, each with its characteristic architecture. The streets were thronged with people, all hurrying somewhere. It was impossible to walk on one's own. You just got in the stream and moved along with it. There were the markets with their wares displayed on the sidewalks, or on rickety stalls which looked ready to collapse at any moment. One store, especially for the tourists, had saris in such profusion and so close to each other that one did not know where to start to look and no one was interested in trying to help. Well! This was new and old Delhi.

We had been in India for five days, when we were to fly to Jaipur. This was an election year and the voting was to occur, whilst we were there. All the Indian airlines were on strike, all emphasising their importance in the hope of gaining a rise in salary. Well, some other form of transportation was needed and our guide – an Indian, now American – finally arranged for two motor coaches to take us there. I was delighted, for now we would see the countryside at first hand and its people and how they live.

Jaipur is the capital of Rajastan, an arid region with camels and elephants for beasts of burden. The countryside was quite fertile. Acres and acres of cultivated land stretched before us. It was the women who were working in the fields, patiently hoeing row by row with hand-held tools. The afternoon was drawing into evening and hordes of men were returning from work, either walking or riding bicycles. The women were slowly making their way back from the fields and, on route, they all stopped at the communal well, filled their terra cotta ollas with water and placed them on their heads to transport them home for the evening meal.

As we drove along the two-laned highway in the gathering dusk, an oncoming truck hit our driver's outside mirror. He just continued on his merry way but our driver, despite almost bumper to bumper traffic, turned the bus around and finally caught up with the truck driver. He made him pull over and stop. Much verbiage followed, but obviously with no resolution. So both men walked down the road to a filling station and were shortly joined by a Holy Man. From what we could see from our seats he became the mediator, but it took a long time before an amicable decision was reached. We could not communicate with our driver because of the language barrier, but we later learned from our guide that the truck driver had to admit to his part in the problem. Unless he did, our driver would be held accountable for the broken mirror and lose his job.

Well, night was drawing on and we still had a long way to go to our hotel. Imagine our surprise when our driver pulled into a very private driveway and we arrived at Samode Palace, the residence of the Maharaja of Jaipur and our home for the next two days and nights. Our journey had been quite an adventure and we were all ready for a drink, a shower and a meal, but this was not to be. For the Maharaja and his wife had arranged a welcome for us that we could not forego. The reception room that we entered, after climbing a long flight of steps, was overwhelmingly elegant and very awe inspiring. We were escorted to our rooms and found an invitation to a cocktail party to meet our host and hostess. Both greeted us graciously and wished us a happy stay. When the last guest had been welcomed, the Maharaja and his wife retired to their private quarters and we were directed to the dining room, where a sumptuous meal was served. Then, we went to bed. No bed had ever been more welcome.

After an elegant English breakfast, the following morning, we set off to explore that interesting area of India. Jaipur was known as the Pink City of Rajastan, because so many of its buildings were painted a lovely soft pink hue. The city was bustling, thronged with people – natives – and, again, the sacred cows mingled with the humans. Again the cattle restricted the traffic. We then visited The Amber Fort, and toured another awe inspiring palace, which we reached by riding on the back of a gaily decorated elephant. The trip was short, thank goodness, that gentle swaying would soon have put me to sleep.

On our seventh day in this continent, we were off to Agra,

settled in our comfortable motor coach again. There was no excitement en route today. We stopped at Fatehpur Sikri, the deserted sandstone city built by Emperor Akbar in the sixteenth century. How well this site had been preserved! Many of the exterior walls were still standing and intact after three hundred years, and the architecture was gracious and soothing. We were all anxious to get to the next stage of our journey, Agra and the Taj Mahal. There it was, in the distance. As we drew closer, that magnificent monument stood out in all its lacy white grandeur and, as we moved to the other side, there it was reflected in the water. Later, when the sun started to set, the whiteness turned into a golden hue that somehow reassured us that tomorrow would be another great day. Yes! I had been right. It was one of the romantic moments of my life. What a wonderful place to be proposed to, I thought. As we started to walk away from the building and through the park, we noticed a throng of young people and that boys walked only with boys and girls walked only with girls. Yes, we were right, our guide told us. It was only when one was affianced that young people were allowed to walk together. Now we took our last look at that wonderful monument. The sun had almost set and it reared its beautiful head to the sky still. Still dimly outlined in the gathering dusk, it conveyed a sense of beauty and also a sense of hope. We said goodbye sadly and hoped to return another year.

The next day was Saturday and we went to Khajuraho. Again, our guide had been able to arrange a motor coach for us. It was a long drive, despite several stops to stretch and to drink. Finally, we arrived at the Oberoi Hotel. After a short rest, we went off to see the erotic and exotic temples built by the Chandela Kings between AD 950 and AD 1050. They were something worth seeing. They were very well preserved and the carving was magnificent. There was certainly nothing like those holy places in the West, but there was a grotesqueness that detracted from the beauty. I guess that this was a cultural factor and may have had a special meaning unknown to us. It was all worth that long coach ride.

Next, we were on our way to Varanasi. No coaches were available and so we had a fleet of small cars with native drivers. Would we make it? we thought. Will we really reach our destination?

Never have I ridden with such drivers. They all drove on the white middle line. When approached by an oncoming car, the driver suddenly jerked his car to the side, sending passengers flying and missing the approaching car by inches! Was this par for the course there, or was the practice just to give us a thrill? I just closed my eyes and kept my fingers crossed and we finally arrived in Varanasi without any mishap. We later learned that this was the way that they drove in this part of the world and I was glad that we did not have many other long trips to face. We returned to New Delhi from Varanasi by train and that, too, was another experience.

Varanasi is the modern name for Benares. It, too, is a bustling town on the Ganges River, and it is here that thousands of Hindus came to the steps to immerse themselves in the Ganges, releasing their souls from reincarnation. The banks of the river were strewn with white shrouded bodies awaiting cremation in the burning ghats and having their ashes dispersed into the river. It was a touching scene, watching the bodies being brought to the river, strapped on top of a small car, then loaded into the burning pyre by family and relatives, all observed by the sacred cows. We sailed on the Ganges. The view of the city was overwhelming and the populace, washing their dirty linen in the river and drying it on the steps, gave an added bizarre feeling to the whole scene. We had been warned not to drink the water from the river. Well, just to look at that water would warn anyone that it was very contaminated. Nevertheless, as we sailed along, we witnessed several families taking their morning bath in the filthy waters. Ugh! let's go home, I thought. All the glamour of the Ganges had been destroyed for me.

We were supposed to fly from Varanasi to Katmandu, but the airline strikes made this impossible. No other means of transportation could get us there and back in time for our flight home. I was really disappointed. For the one place that I really wanted to see and enjoy was Everest. We were carried back to New Delhi by train and this gave us a chance to see some aspects of urban and suburban life, as we travelled by towns and villages with their houses and hovels and communal facilities. I bought a cup of tea at one of the station stops, served in a small terracotta bowl. It was just like drinking soup. Others on the train broke their little bowl. It was not good to reuse it. I still have mine and use it for flowers, a happy memento of a very different vacation in a very different part of the world. As always it was good to get home and back to our routine. Once again, we settled back and life resumed and went on.

1990

The holidays came and went with the usual festivities, but nothing really changed in our relationship, despite Hank's continuing in therapy. The winter passed and, with the arrival of spring, Esther and Colin announced their intention to marry. This was most exciting, despite my belief that Colin needed to grow and mature some if he was to enjoy his role as head of the house. Everything fell into place and, on 8 September, my mother's birthday, they were joined in wedlock before their friends and family in a quiet ceremony at Littleworth Farm. It was a happy day for all of us, despite Hank's lack of improvement and a new turn of events. He had returned from one of his therapy sessions saying that he was now going into analysis. It was the only avenue left to him.

'That will be the end of our marriage,' I said.

'Well, it's a risk that I have to take,' was his reply.

He had given no thought to the consequences for anyone else, and said that he could no longer continue to live with the situation as it was. How was it? As usual we had no discussion or comments. He said that he was now experiencing panic attacks, but I had never seen these at home. Then he started to have terrible nightmares and became overwhelmed with fears and anxieties whenever it was time to go to sleep. One night, I awoke to a sobbing sound and found him in the bathroom with his razor. I quickly removed it and called his analyst and, after talking with him for some time, Hank settled down. I didn't go to sleep and I had no one to help me with my own anxiety.

As he regressed, in the early stages of his analysis, life became more and more difficult. We still could not talk about his problem, and I never knew what this was. I had no access to his therapist, who refused to discuss my husband's problem with me under the guise of confidentiality between patient and physician.

Once the excitement of the wedding was over we settled again into a no man's land, each doing his own thing. How lucky I was to have a job to which I could give myself. I spent a great deal of my time involved in one or other professional activity.

As 1991 progressed, I again wanted to get away for a while and a cruise down the River Danube was presented to me. It was just what I wanted. I had sailed on many of the large rivers of the world and now here was a chance to sail on one more. We went, despite the war in Yugoslavia and, again, we spent a wonderful three weeks on that boat. During this trip, I decided that we had to get some communication going. We couldn't go on in such isolation but I failed, as on so many other occasions. We had only been home a short time, when Hank returned from his daily session demanding a divorce. He had found out from his analyst that we could separate for a given period, that this separation could be within the same house, and a no-fault divorce could be had without either of us attending court. In essence, our lawyers could fix it all up for us. How did his therapist know so much about it all? I thought. He wasn't a lawyer. Well, he was having his own mid-life crisis and they were working on the same kind of things. The separation did not materialise. Week after week went by, and Hank was still sharing the downstairs rooms with me, despite our agreeing that he would move upstairs and care for himself. Finally, I asked if he was still interested in this plan, or had things changed? Slowly, that weekend, he moved himself and his belongings upstairs, but he continued to eat with me. When I asked my lawyer about this, he said that I was entitled to my privacy and, after that, the separation was effected.

Separation

1 January 1993

By 1 January 1993, Hank and I had been separated within the same house – 428 N Essex – for the past ten months. He had been in analysis for the past four years. The separation was at his request and as a result of deciding in his analysis what was right for him. No consideration was given to the needs of other family members, and no thought was given to the consequences of his behaviour.

He announced to the world – his family and a few friends – 'Pat and I are splitting,' as though this was an everyday occurrence. There was no sorrow or unhappiness, only a jolliness and sense of satisfaction and accomplishment. He was totally surprised by my feelings of anger, of being cheated and betrayed. We had been married for more than thirty years, but those years were erased from his mind and thinking.

Despite our differences, I never thought or expected to be faced with this challenge. I now had to cope with the unhappiest time of my life. This was what the profession called a 'narcissistic slap in the face'. I felt furious, degraded and demeaned. I was alone, lonely and desolate but, out of all this misery, I came to realise who my friends were, and who were the most important people in my life. I appreciated the devotion of Esther and Colin, and Mary and Jim.

With the help of Sally, Doe and Wira, I passed through all the stages of anger; the victim stage, indignation stage, survivor stage, and I tried to reorganise my life. I had wonderful friends, but who was my very, very, best friend – 'that damned dog,' to quote Hank – Oliver! He never let me down. He was always there – a joy and a comfort in my hour of need. He was a true friend!

Ollie was Esther's dog and came to me when she could no longer care for him because of her work schedule. We knew each other well and he was the nicest dog that I had ever had. We understood each other's vibes and he became my shadow. He knew when I was happy, he knew when I was sad and he always responded with appropriate feelings, talking to me with his tail or tongue. Yes, Ollie was my salvation. Was he sent to us for this? I thought. For he was a stray and found his own way into our lives and our hearts. His caring and devotion carried me through that desolate time.

Looking back over these unhappy times, I saw that it was because of them that I began to see the true Hank. I had never really looked beneath that conforming, ingratiating exterior. There was nothing there that I could admire. Yes! Dad was right. He had described him as undisciplined, unable to accept responsibility for himself and his behaviour, unprincipled, unable to take a stand. Now after all those years together, I saw him as callow (no guts), callous (no empathy), controlling (getting his own way no matter what the consequences) and conniving. Now, I realise that he aroused pity in me. Was this the reason that I had married him? Was that what had kept us together? My most recent reading, *Husbands Who Won't Lead* by James Walker, confirmed my feelings and fears. He identified the passive resistive male – typically Hank – and identified several categories, the most severe being the escapist and his quest for fantasy and pleasure to deaden the pain of defeat and avoid the sense of disrespect. His hallmark was chronic irresponsibility. Well with all that increased understanding, where had it got me?

Initially, I did not want a divorce. I had hoped that we could work together, to solve whatever our problems were and spend long weekends together at Littleworth, alone or with our friends. That was the reason for acquiring the farm, wasn't it? The analyst knocked this idea on the head. Of course, he didn't want to lose his five hundred dollars a week fee, and Hank said he did not want to be back down there with me! Ah, there it was. He obviously had no feelings left for me. So we had better get on with the sordid affair, I thought.

To emphasise my need to be free, just as much as he needed it, I told him to take care of his own needs, including his laundry. His ambivalence continued. He did not do any of the things that we had agreed to. So I (here we go again) finally arranged a meeting with Hank and his lawyer at my lawyer's office in the hopes of getting on with the legal separation. I continued in limbo because of his ambivalence. Very soon now, I would be on my way to Jamaica for three months, February, March and April, where I would work with the child psychiatrist, Pauline Milbourne MD under a UNICEF grant.

Before I left, I made some concrete plans for my return. After visiting White Horse Village where my friend Sally lived, I decided to buy into the co-operative. They would have an apartment waiting for me on my return. I could leave for warmer climes with a sense of settlement. Once again, I had been the one to find a positive solution to our problems but, alas, I had once again fallen into his trap, my acting out of his ambivalence and giving him the ability to project the problem on to me and make it look like it was my fault. Well never mind, some resolution had to be made and I could leave with peace of mind and a future to look forward to.

One more decision had to be made before I left. What did I want out of all this mess? I wanted to keep Littleworth Farm for Esther, as well as myself. It represented all of my Englishness. This was agreeable to Hank, who was glad that I did not want the Narberth House. He did not want to move and really couldn't if he was to continue in analysis, as he was planning to do. He suggested that I should talk to my lawyer, who then arranged all the legal aspects of our taking the house of our choice. Hank signed the agreement, before I left for Jamaica.

I would return a free woman, move into White Horse Village and acquire Littleworth Farm. The arrival of my English inheritance was timely, arriving in my American bank at a welcome time. What a joy to look forward to, away from his sickness with its control and manipulation. My lawyer, ever shrewd as lawyers are, helped me to see that even though my actions were my usual patterns of 'Patsy to the rescue', this time, it was also my way of taking care of me. What of my very best friend, Ollie? Colin's mother offered to care for him during my absence. Now I knew that he would be loved and well cared for. He would be among his friends, too, I could leave, knowing that all was under control and with a peaceful mind.

It was 30 January 1993 and I awaited the taxi to take me to the airport and my flight to Miami and Kingston, Jamaica.

Jamaica, British West Indies, February to April 1993

In February 1993, we touched down not in Kingston but in Montego Bay, or Mo'bay as the natives knew it. As I made my way to the exit, an elderly Jamaican male approached me. He enquired who I was. Then he took my luggage and escorted me to his minibus. I got to know that man and his bus very well for I and the students rode in it daily, to and from the clinic. He took me to the Courtleigh Hotel, where a pleasant one bedroom apartment awaited me. He arranged to meet me there the next day at half past eight to take me to the clinic. Well there I was in Jamaica. I felt that I would like the capital, Kingston, with its old and new quarters. What a wonderful opportunity awaited me! Was I not lucky to have been chosen to participate in a venture sponsored by AACAP? Was I not lucky that the clinic at home gave me three months leave of absence to allow me to accept?

It was still quite early and I wandered around to get my bearings. The hotel was an attractive modern building, set amidst palms and enormous mango trees. There was a swimming pool just outside my apartment building, and another closer to the main building. Beside this pool there was an attractive gazebo, with which I became very familiar as it served informal but tasty meals at very attractive prices. The grounds were set way back from the main highway which, at this time, was still very busy with buses and private cars bumper to bumper as the locals wended their way home after a busy day. The following day I would join that bustling throng. Beyond the road the mountains could be seen soaring upwards. They seemed indistinct and hazy, but something to explore at another time. Time was marching on and I was hungry. I sampled my first meal of chicken jerky in the gazebo. It was good and there were many more good meals in the weeks ahead. I returned to my temporary home and bed.

The next day, the Jamaica experience began. I found several young women in the hotel lobby and they, too, moved toward the bus as it pulled up to the door. They were some of the students that I was there to teach. They, too, had an apartment, not too far from mine. Each one was from a different Caribbean Island, Antigua, Dominica, St Lucia, and St Vincent. The other students whom we met shortly were from Jamaica, and most of them were from Kingston. We entered the bus and were transported to the clinic. We passed through a business district and were soon in a rather poverty-stricken neighbourhood. Property was shabby and even derelict. We entered a compound surrounded by high concrete walls, through gates guarded by two men in uniform who allowed us to enter only after talking for some time with our driver. Was this a prison? I thought. No, it was a complex of medical buildings and offices. Why was there so much protection? I wondered. After a few days we were admitted without question.

We reached the clinic building and we were greeted by the Director, Dr Pauline Milbourne. She was a native Jamaican who did her psychiatry training at Hahnneman University in Philadelphia. She knew of me by name, but had not been able to participate in my school programme because of the cut in our funding. She found work for all the students and then she and I discussed how I hoped that we could approach our challenge. The reports on the following pages give the reader some idea of the curriculum, and so I could focus on the other and more social side of those three months.

As we travelled back and forth in the bus, I got to know the other students well. They were a friendly group and, as the days and weeks went by, we became good friends. We soon realised that we were all avid tourists and after our 'clinic day' we were anxious to explore our new environment. Best of all, I was always included in their adventures. We participated in as many local events and occasions as we could and we met many interesting people. The most touching incident of our day-to-day living was the arrival of a stray dog with her very new puppy. Stray dogs were everywhere in that poverty stricken neighbourhood, but that one had a pup and had found the shelter of the campus, perhaps after being fed by the gatekeepers. We soon endeared ourselves to them and they to us, and we saved scraps from our evening meal to offer to them for breakfast.

They began to watch for our bus to arrive and they welcomed us as we alighted from the vehicle, knowing that something good was forthcoming. How could we not feed those little orphans? we asked ourselves. Most of the locals paid no attention to them. Soon the mother dog became aware of our trip to the cafeteria for lunch and she and her pup would be waiting for our exit, hoping for more refreshment. We never said no! The dogs followed us back to the clinic. We pooled our scraps and they lapped everything up. This became part of our daily routine. The dogs stayed close to the clinic through the afternoon and, as our bus pulled away at the day's end, they pathetically moved toward the gates. Where they spent the nights and weekends we never knew, but they were always waiting the next day. I used the mother dog's maternal behaviour to emphasise the human infant's needs and the maternal behaviour these elicited and the students remarked on how helpful our romance with the animals had been. As my professor once said, 'It behoves a teacher to use any and every avenue to get his point across,' and so I did.

Sightseeing in Jamaica

January 1993 was a very mild month in the USA. February was anything but. Snow and blizzards made the news. Again, how lucky I was to be away, but my heart went out to my friends and family and I encouraged them to come and stay with me in Jamaica, just to escape the winter misery. Nobody refused, and so, as each came, we visited all these places that I had discovered and enjoyed.

Kingston itself was a very attractive city with its coastline backed by the verdant Blue Mountains. So this was where we usually started our explorations. Kingston was built around the seventh largest natural harbour in the world. The Saint William Grant Park was truly spectacular. Port Royal, on the harbour, the most famous place in the Caribbean, grew enormously wealthy on plunder and became known as 'the wickedest city in the world'. Uptown, we enjoyed Devon House, built in the 1880s as a millionaire's residence with its shopping and restaurant complex. At that time of year, the gardens were exotic with the tropical flora in full bloom. One shrub of cleradendron made me homesick for my plant, but mine would never be as beautiful as this one in Kingston.

The botanical gardens were again overwhelming with their profusion of tropical flora and foliage, but the house that I liked best was King's House, the official residence of the governor general because of its British architecture. The major point of interest though, was the Bob Marley Museum, a name that I had no acquaintance with until my stay in Jamaica. The Blue Mountains were also one of my favourite places and they got their name from the hues that we saw as we looked towards them in the early morning or later afternoon light. The national tree was the blue mahoe, but the mountain slopes were covered with mahogany, satinwood, cedar, Spanish elm and many other trees whose names I did not remember. All were used in furniture making and for fine craft items. Breadfruit, coconut and mangoes were also prolific. I was enamoured with the native and imported species of orchids, something that I had enjoyed growing at home.

Spanish Town, not too far a drive from Kingston, was my kind of town, old, old, old. It was Jamaica's first capital and was founded in 1534. The old town square gave it real ambience and there were many places of historical interest around it. One of the best ways to see Jamaica was to drive from Kingston to Montego Bay, the tourist resort on the north coast. Nevertheless, there was much of historical interest to see in the town, and the drive back along the northern coastline gave one a sense of the whole island.

The trip that I and all my friends enjoyed most was the one to Saint Elizabeth and the Black River safari. Gliding down the river, we were very soon in a mangrove swamp. Never had any of us seen its like before. The water was filled with aquatic plants which had a beautiful purple blossom, as well as water lilies which were just beginning to flower. The mangroves hung down into the water like graceful curtains and, sleeping under these, there were crocodiles of all sizes. The reflection of the sun on the water was unbelievable. No words could describe it and even our photographs did not convey the reality of those experiences.

Nobody left Jamaica disappointed. The weather for the winter weary Americans was a tonic and the cuisine was acceptable and enjoyed by all my friends. The one aspect that we all commented on was the wonderful blending of the historical with nature. Nobody said goodbye without saying that they would be back soon.

Return from Jamaica

I returned on 28 April 1993. Jamaica was just what I had needed, away from the stress and tension of life in Philadelphia. I had time to think of what I needed and how to achieve it. The settlement with Hank went well – 'as these things go,' said my lawyer. But Hank gave himself away when I raised the question of what he planned to do with the boat, which he had not declared in his assets. Both lawyers were annoyed. Both had some fantasy that this was a huge expensive yacht! When they learned that it was only a small whaler, they were somewhat appeased and again when Hank agreed to give it to Esther and Colin.

Now I owned Littleworth Farm and ten acres as well as my little apartment at White Horse Village. I came out of that mess quite well, but I thought of all that I had invested in our living over those thirty years. Now Ollie and I were finally settled into a pleasant routine – Saturday, Sunday, Monday and Tuesday in Maryland, and Wednesday, Thursday and Friday in Pennsylvania. I could continue to work at the clinic on a part-time basis and this suited me fine. It gave meaning and focus to my life. The following week, I went to Santa Fe and then on to Portland, Oregon, to meet with Dick Olmsted and report on my experience in Jamaica.

After reading Scott Peck's book, *People of the Lie*, I understood Hank's problem much better and recognised how sick he was due to his self-devaluation and inability to let himself be loved. I remember how I had diagnosed that three months into marriage. Now I realised that the divorce may have been the best thing that had happened to me. At least I was free to follow whatever path opened up.

White Horse Village, 12 May 1993 to 1 April 1997

Everything was arranged and I moved into White Horse Village on 12 May 1993, less than two weeks after arriving back from Jamaica. Sally had made the arrangements with the movers and they arrived at eight o'clock. The previous evening I had told

Hank that they would be there and his immediate response was, 'Have them bring my things from Littleworth back here.' He was totally floored when I said that was not where I was moving to. Anyway, when Ollie and I visited the farm the next weekend, his belongings had been moved out. That was one less problem to solve for him.

Now my very best friend and I were comfortably settled in Apartment 138, a studio garden apartment that was comfortable, quiet and peaceful and it was all mine. The furnishings fitted nicely, and gave an ambience of my English home. The sliding doors opened onto a nice patio, which I filled with flowers and on which I hung a feeder for the birds. One afternoon, several months after I had moved in, I was surprised to see a rose breasted grosbeak enjoying his meal on the feeder, a bird that I had not seen before, or since. The neighbours were friendly and it was certainly nice to have one's evening meal ready and available, either informally in the coffee shop, or formally in the dining room, or even available to take home and eat, whenever and however one was inclined. The best part for me was the feeling of safety and security, something I had never thought about before but now, as a single older woman, something I needed to overcome was my sense of vulnerability and insecurity.

Life returned to its usual routines. I continued to work and my social life was once again on track. Wira lived close by and we arranged to spend Wednesday evenings together. Whenever there was an activity at White Horse Village – and there were many – she would join me to participate whenever she could. This gave an outlet for her, for she was caring for her aged mother and was very house bound, even though she did have good sitters available when needed. We enjoyed the trips that were arranged for us. We went to the Flower Show very easily by bus, which was also waiting for us on our exiting. We made trips to the orchestra in Philadelphia, again with door to door transportation, to the local theatres, to Longwood Gardens, and to localities further afield in New Jersey, Delaware and Pennsylvania. We had movies every Friday night, and always something special at holiday times. We were spoilt, and we shamelessly enjoyed being spoilt.

Single Again, 1994

New Beginnings

Life went on! The divorce was finalised by the lawyers and, on 13 July 1993, I was now one of the hordes of single – and lonely – women. It was embarrassing and humiliating to admit that one was alone. I had not wanted to sever our marriage. Rather, I had wanted to know the problem and work together with Hank to solve it, but this was against all the rules of analysis. The problem would never be revealed and, so, the profession that had been so good to me had now betrayed me and let me down.

Well, again I must count my blessings and get on with my life and I did. Just after the finalisation, Wira and Sally met with me for dinner and although we could not consider it a festive occasion, there was a sense that something had ended and something was about to begin. So we drank to the present and to what the future would bring. After being resident for more than three years at White Horse Village, I had an attack of poison ivy which made itself known on a Saturday morning. I raced to the physician's office, for previous experience had told me that to delay was dangerous. I was told, in no uncertain terms, that I could not be seen for four days. No alternative was suggested. Only I knew now allergic I was to poison ivy, and there no one wanted to know! I could not wait. For me, this was just as urgent as a heart attack. I needed help, and I needed it then. This was why I was living there, to be physically as well as mentally safe. I jumped into the car and drove to the emergency room at Bryn Mawr Hospital, where I was promptly and adequately treated in what I knew was the right way.

Nobody at White Horse Village responded to my complaints, neither the administration nor the physician, and I began to have second thoughts about how this organisation was fulfilling its promises. I began to realise that I really did not fit into the social milieu. I was next to the youngest occupant. I still worked and, although I did enjoy the activities, I could arrange those for myself. In any event I was only there for three days a week. I was at Littleworth more than I was there.

For the past two years I had known Len, a neighbour on the Neck in Cambridge. We enjoyed each other's company and spent time together when we could. He had been widowed for two years and was still recovering from his loss. We were both grieving. I think I brought a new spark into his life, as he did into mine. He had tried a retirement home in Easton and didn't like the regimentation. He had moved to Chatham Village in Easton, just twelve miles from Cambridge for a haven from the icy winters and the hot and humid summers. That's just what I wanted too. So we decided to become 'partners' and share a two-bedroomed and two bath apartment in the Village. We would be together, and yet we would be apart and free to manage our farms as we were needed. So, on 1 April 1997, in the worst snowstorm experienced on the east coast, I packed my belongings and Ollie and I moved south. A new life was to begin, and I prayed that the snowstorm did not auger the shape of things to come.

The Writing Class

The writing class was my entrance into Easton society. I was warmly welcomed by all the participants and on my second session I decided to write a poem to usher in a new life, just a simple poem, *The Optimist*, but this was my first writing effort apart from professional papers that I read before a live audience. Then the writing session was over and the summer vacation stretched before us. During this lull in life's tempo, I began to think seriously of writing my autobiography and I finally identified the purpose and how I wanted to do it. The reason for doing it was purely for me to learn how I came to be me. I would review my life and express my thoughts and feelings through the written word. Hopefully, I could be objective and express my perceptions whether these were, in reality, right or wrong. I decided to start at the beginning and slowly let my life evolve, using each developmental phase to focus my personal growth. For wasn't growth what life was all about? I would see how nature and nurture had worked together on my behalf. I must see how I could convey this, fairly and honestly.

Mark Twain described an autobiography as, 'the truest of all books. For while it inevitably consists mainly of extinctions of truth, shirkings of truth, partial revealments of the truth, with hardly an instance of plain straight truth, the remorseless truth was there between the lines'.

I decided to try to stick strictly to the truth as I perceived it. When the fall session began, I joined the group which now met at Londonderry – a retirement village which loaned us their library for the two hours that we met – on Thursdays from one o'clock to three o'clock. There were several people in the group whom I remembered, the Baynhams – Leonard and Dorsey both of whom had been kind to me and whom, I later learned, had lived in Wales for several years. Dorsey was especially helpful to me through the group discussions, as I struggled to develop my authorship. Another couple – the Hamiltons, Ralph and Amelia – could not have been more supportive with both their praise and constructive criticism. The group was overseen by Lila, an author with published books to her credit, who encouraged the group to express their comments about each reading, and who added the final touches to these critiques.

Not only did we work and write together, but we also socialised too. At the end of each six week session, we had a pot luck luncheon at which we enjoyed and critiqued each other's culinary feats. Then, one evening, a Saturday I think, we all went to the Church Hill Playhouse to see a former group member play the lead in *The Last of the Red Hot Lovers*. Dinner and the show somehow amalgamated the group and we all seemed to be more friendly and more free with each other.

At the end of my first year, Len decided that he had developed as far as he wanted to and so I continued with the group alone. Each new session brought new people, as well as a coterie of older members. It was with this latter group that I felt a closeness developing. During our sessions, I was always amazed at the variety of experiences that members shared. Backgrounds were varied and many were quite colourful. Family values and mores were extremely disparate. Yet there was an empathy that was difficult to define. All of us had experienced sorrow and happiness, and we cried together and laughed together as we relived each other's life journey.

As the weeks passed, we could see the growth in each other's writing methods and techniques. Imagery was so well expressed that we were transported to the scene; feelings were so well expressed that we readily empathised with them. Historical data and facts were lucidly described and relationships were seen as both supportive or not, as the case may be. When the group functioned effectively – when it was motivated to achieve its goal – and when most members were supportive of each other, I personally felt that I was with caring friends. I left, determined to keep on writing and returned the following week with readable material, no matter how difficult the task. Exposing thoughts and feelings could be difficult, but there were times when socialisation and chatter, even if autobiographical, became predominant. Time was wasted and those – me in particular – who wanted the input from the group felt utterly frustrated. I would have preferred to spend the time writing more of my saga. Yes, narcissistic me, but, after all, my autobiography had to cover a long lifetime and time was marching on!

After eighteen months with the group, my life's story was taking shape and form. Now, how would I present all this information? I wondered. Well, in book form – how else? Thanks to Len's generosity, I had the loan of his old electric typewriter and I now typed, rather than recorded by longhand, all these salient facts that would add up in the end and show me how I came to be me.

New Friends

Before I had moved permanently to the eastern shore, I met a neighbour on Ross Neck Road who was the president of ASK (Activities Singles Klub). He knew Len, who had been a member of the Klub, and he invited us to the numerous picnics that the members organised throughout the summer. We rejoined the Klub and became part of a motley group. We socialised as often as we could and associations developed and slowly grew into friendships. We enjoyed many good meals and camaraderie, as we got to know each other. Lou and Barb became part of our social scene, dining together and theatre going as the occasion arose. Just after I had moved to Chatham Village, one of our neighbours introduced herself. She and her husband were Pennsylvanians and so we were on common ground. She invited me to accompany her to the AAUW summer picnic at the Easton Club. Of course I did and shortly afterwards I became a member, too. Nobody could have been more welcoming than the president, Kay W, and nobody could have made more effort to include me in the ongoing activities. I was still a very new and unknown member to many of the members but I was greatly touched at the last meeting when one of the attendees sought me out to ask how Mary was, following her recent head injury after falling from a horse and that lady had met me only twice. She reminded me that I was leaving for Santa Fe right after the last meeting. What a good memory she had.

Perhaps no one else has had such an experience but, a few weeks ago, ASK and AAUW had meetings on the same night. Both meetings were held in private homes on the same street, only five doors away from each other. I didn't get to both meetings for I got so involved with the one I was attending that, before I knew it, it was ten o'clock and we were still talking. Perhaps one of the greatest joys of my new life had been in meeting and getting to know Len's son and daughter-in-law and their little girls who were rapidly growing and maturing, and his daughter and her husband. No family could have been kinder and more willing to include me in their family togetherness. Once again, an old adage came to mind, this time from Dr Ross at PCGC who said, 'If you want to stay young at heart, stay attached to the young and growing.' Again, it was another true truth.

I had been welcomed by Len's old friends, Mike and Lorraine, in St Michael's, whom we saw whenever their busy schedule allowed, Al and Lorraine in Naples, Florida and the Neshamkins in Orlando, Florida. We saw these Floridians yearly when we spent some time in Florida ourselves. We shared good food, good cheer and good talk with all of them. It was amazing how much there was to be said after one year. Sadly, all of us were suffering physically but, nonetheless, all of us were managing to enjoy life as it came along.

Last, but not least, was Lily (Lilija, really,) my roommate on a Vantage trip to Europe, at Christmas time. We met and clicked and we have shared many happy hours together since the trip visiting each other in Chatham Village and in upstate New York. Lily was an avid gardener and had always wanted to go to the Philadelphia Flower Show, but had never got there. Well, that was easy to solve. I had always wanted to visit Watkin's Glen and Mark Twain's county and never made it and, once again, that was taken care of too. Yes, the years rolled by, but I did not complain. My life still had more joys than sorrows and I hoped that it would keep going on.

One Weekend in the Country

I now belonged to that august body of human beings who were living in their golden years. I had always supposed that, at that stage of life, one had encountered and coped with most social challenges and had achieved a feeling of self-competence and security. That was not quite true for I had recently been presented with a new and interesting challenge. My very best friend and I were invited to spend the weekend with long-standing and good friends of the former. I had met these people very casually and very briefly, so briefly that I believe that all we had said to each other was, 'Hi,' across a very crowded room. So it was with mixed feelings and much trepidation that I packed a few casual clothes and embarked on the journey.

The friends, whom I will call Bill and Jane, lived in the southern part of Pennsylvania's beautiful Chester County. The trip there was simple and easy. We drove comfortably along super highways until we had passed Newark, Delaware. Then the road became a small country highway, traversing beautiful rolling farm and woodland scenery. It was a joy in itself. We arrived in the area much too early, but we found a pleasant restaurant and enjoyed a home style country lunch. We slowly meandered around until we found their house.

This was an old stone farmhouse, set back from the road within its own rolling acres. A huge stone barn stood close to the house. The sun shone and the locality gave us a warm and friendly welcome. As we neared the house, a host of cats arrived and formed a welcoming committee on the stoop. As we parked the car, our host joined us, greeting us with a merry welcoming smile. He helped me, alight with old world charm and courtesy, and led us to the house. Our hostess was awaiting us, with her own special greeting which included a big bear hug. Scenes of our arrival at Grandmother's house during my childhood flashed before me and I knew that we were indeed very welcome. Before we knew it, we were seated at the dining room table with tea and coffee, gasping at the magnificent country panorama spread before us. We watched the antics of the birds flocking on the feeders and without any of us having spoken very much, I felt at home with people whom I hardly knew. Slowly, we began to realise what our friends had been doing over the few years that they had been together. They had found a farm property which satisfied their needs for togetherness, solitude and contentment. They had restored it, maintaining the ambience of the early nineteenth century but they had added all the modern conveniences necessary for comfort. There was no clutter of modern life. Everything was orderly and neat. There was a place for everything and everything was in its place. Everything and everywhere gleamed and sparkled in the sunny rooms. Every piece of furniture was just right for its location. Nature was also part of the house's interior. Every window ledge recessed in the eighteen inch thick, stone walls held a healthy plant, a fern or a cactus. Despite a busy and hectic work schedule, life in the farmhouse was simple, uncluttered and uncontaminated. It was a wonderful haven from the confusion and chaos of everyday life.

Television was absent, but music and literature had a special place in the house. Our friends' happiness and pleasure seemed to spring from their involvement with the soil and with each other. As we sat in the sun-drenched dining room with its blooming plants and the birds hovering on the feeders outside, and as we gazed at the peaceful rolling scenery, we began to feel a sense of peace and contentment and a feeling that 'All's right with the world'. Is this what was meant by solitude? I thought.

As the soporific feeling became more intense, I began to realise that I was communing with nature, through the flora and fauna, contact with the earth and the sky and even through the orderliness of the grazing animals and the silence. Someone once said that silence in the country was deafening, but not so this silence. It began to cover me like a blanket at first, then began to seep through my body. What relaxation it was. I began to realise what I had missed for so many years. All this peace had been buried under urban and suburban mania, with the confusion, disturbance, conflicts, abrasiveness and aggression. Everything here was in harmony, with a sense of peace on earth, goodwill to men.

As I absorbed the rural atmosphere, I began to discover Bill and Jane. Although Jane was twenty years my junior, this age difference went unnoticed. We clicked spontaneously and found ourselves being drawn closer, sharing similar thoughts, ideas and values. We disagreed on little. She had grown up on a farm and was a true country woman. She loved this farm. It was hers and, no matter what, she was going to spend the rest of her life there and die on this property. Although she had lived on many farms, this one was, and always would be, her true home.

Our host, a European who arrived in the USA in the sixties, still kept in touch with his family and maintained his European ideas and values. He, too, felt the farmhouse was his real home. Both had had stormy previous lives. They had been divorced twice. It now felt as though they had at last found each other. The warmth, contentedness and happiness which radiated from both the man and woman seemed to confirm this. They seemed to mirror the ambience of the locality. They seemed to fit right in with the plain people. They were down to earth, embedded and rooted in nature. They seemed to be just another extension of her practical and purposeful milieu. Nothing was superficial or artificial. Nothing indicated a need to keep up with the Jones'. Nothing was neglected or shabby, nor was there anything extraneous, opulent or ostentatious. Their peace and contentment sprang from this togetherness with nature.

As always, all good times came to an end and so did our weekend. As we said goodbye, a feeling of sadness flooded me. What an experience it had been, to have shared such empathy with two human beings who had been almost strangers. How much I would miss this togetherness. Would we meet again? I hoped so and I hoped that we would get to know each other on a deeper level. As we travelled back to Maryland, a feeling of contentment and fulfilment over came me and raised many questions. What made these two people, both younger than I and with whom I had little in common, like me and so quickly accept me as a friend and vice versa? I asked myself. What vibes did we feel from each other that made us feel that we had known each other for more than the few hours that we were together? I wished that I knew! This weekend has reinforced for me my belief that human beings were affected by their interest in, and willingness to live with, nature. As I recalled the writings of Wordsworth, Hardy, the Brontes, they all expressed their belief that the joys of nature were the essence of life. My experience this weekend had convinced me that this is true.

I too was truly a country girl, with basic country values. Yes, layers of urbanisation and suburbanisation had accumulated. Now they were slowly being shed. No longer did I have great material wants or needs. I was happy to enjoy simpler aspects of life, provided that I had the company of friends whom I had known for more than half a lifetime. As I looked back over the years, I realised that a de-urbanising process had been festering within me, a process started almost twenty years ago. It was then that we acquired our little Dorchester County farm. Now I knew how important this was to me and why I would never let it go.

Poughkeepsie Revisited

In June 1998 we went to a surprise fiftieth birthday party in Albany, New York, for my friend's daughter. Since we would be passing close to Poughkeepsie, we decided to revisit the area which welcomed me to the USA. It was a gorgeous day. Brilliant sunshine was reflected from the river, as we crossed the Mid Hudson Bridge. Here we were! The sign said, 'City of Poughkeepsie'. We kept following the traffic. Nothing looked familiar but then a signpost pointed to our right saying 'Vassar College'.

We decided to find our motel first, check in and then get our bearings. There was the motel, just as they had said, at the junction of the roads. Again, nothing looked familiar. We were put on course by the motel keeper and arrived without any difficulty at the college. This area did look somewhat as I remembered it.

Cars were parked and a few people were walking on the campus. The summer school had not yet started.

'Now, let's see if we can get downtown,' I said.

Nothing looked familiar but we followed our noses and we did come to Main Street. What had happened? Every building was boarded up. Poughkeepsie, as most American towns and cities, had moved into the twentieth century and had replaced downtown with shopping malls throughout the urban area. The one we visited was, indeed, a shoppers' paradise, but where was the ambience of the old city centre?

'Now, let's find the hospital,' I suggested. We wound back and forth through the streets and finally found it. Again, I had another shock! There was nothing here that I remembered. The original building had been added to and our one hundred and fifty year old original structure had been lost in the huge modern extension attached to it. Nothing of that stately façade was left. Building was still in progress and I wondered how so much addition was needed in this era of limited hospital care. Of course, Vassar Brother's Hospital served a large area, but then so did St Francis, its rival, and this seemed not to have changed at all. What had happened to the road on which we used to walk to town? I thought. I remembered those early days of my stay when I walked to the Post Office just for fresh air and exercise, and my irritation when a hospital employee would offer me a lift into the town. Later, as I became Americanised, how irritated I got with them if they didn't stop and offer me the same lift! This time I never turned it down.

A new building had been erected and the sign proclaimed that it was to be a Drug Rehabilitation Centre, clearly a sign of our times! We drove along the Hudson's eastern shore, on Route Nine. There was nothing familiar. Several malls had replaced the verdant countryside. All seemed to be booming. The Marist College was still as I recalled but there was a new building, The Culinary Institute of America, which added another college to Poughkeepsie's credit, making it an educational as well as a vacation centre. It was still the home of IBM.

The tourist attractions, Hyde Park, Roosevelt's home, and the Vanderbilt Mansion looked just the same. I must come back to

Poughkeepsie and get reacquainted, and re-explore Duchess County in all its new and unfamiliar glory, Red Hook and Rhinebeck to the north, Wappinger's Falls, Beekman and Poughquag to the south, and Pleasant Valley. Had it continued to live up to its name? Despite those happy years that I spent there, I felt like an alien in a strange land! Fall was beautiful in the Catskills, so I decided to select a date to return to this idyllic county of New York State and relive some of its pleasures then. Now I had my own car and time to spare and I did not believe that nature would let me down.

Depression and More Sadness and Sorrow

It was a beautiful day for the time of year, 7 January 1999. The sky was azure blue and the sun poured down, but my mood did not mirror the world outside. I had felt 'down' for some time now, all related I believed to Esther's news of the pending separation from Colin. My heart bled for them, not so much that they were not happy together, for this could be righted, especially at their age, but for fear that they were experiencing that terrible feeling of failure which overcame me when Hank told me that he wanted a divorce. Hopefully, their feelings were mitigated by the fact that they could talk about their differences and there seemed to be no anger or hostility between them. There was no discussion for me, no reason offered, only that Hank's therapist – analyst – had helped him to decide what was right for him, but on what basis? There was no answer. What about what was right for the family? Did he not have responsibilities to the children if not to his wife?

Well, today I was down and blue, blue, blue. I had never felt so low. Why? I asked myself. Was this what was meant by depression? I felt alone, alienated from everything and everyone, useless and hopeless. Well, whatever, I must get on. I needed to get the chores out of the way. Ginny was coming and we'd have a good lunch, catch up on our activities and then see the group at the writing class. For Lila had promised a make-up class today, partly out of her own need, as she reminded us that she would not have seen us for three weeks and she would be lonely after the holidays.

Oh! and don't forget the dinner date at half past five with the

Mental Health Association at Channel Markers, I thought. Come on, it's going to be an interesting day, I tried to convince myself, and I would be going to Philadelphia at the weekend. I finished the crossword puzzle and there was Ginny, dressed warmly and gaily in a soft blue, Chinese style outfit, just what I would like. We caught up on all the news and went over to Londonderry. Well! we were the first. It was not yet one o'clock. We settled in the room and continued our gossiping. Still no one showed. It was half past one and still we were alone. What had happened? We went back to Chatham and called Lila, who claimed she was sick and had been for the past ten days. She had been too ill to call us, but she had called Bob. She was surprised that he had not called us. He had called everyone else. Well it was no great disaster. I shared some thoughts with Ginny about writing techniques. We reviewed some of Montgomery's *Anne of Green Gables* series and she gave me some good advice regarding Joey's painting. She told me to take it to Troika and have it framed to give it protection. She left and I made myself ready for the dinner.

On arriving, I was greeted with friendliness and inclusion. I felt as though I was amongst old friends, although I have never met those people before. Anyway this was an exciting time to be in Talbot County, with its mental health plans and the emphasis on child mental health. I was asked if I would participate. Of course I would, but how? I asked. We would see, I was told. Right then, they were going to implement Berry Brazelton's Touch Point programme and they wanted me to be part of it. So we arranged to meet at Londonderry on Monday, 11 January for breakfast and I would begin to sort out who was who and what was what. Best of all, there was to be a family and children's programme developed along the way and I might just have what that was going to take.

What had happened? I thought. I no longer felt blue and down as I got ready for bed. Of course I didn't. I had been recognised as someone with talent and needed skills and openly welcomed into a group without having to prove myself first. Again, I now have something to live for, something that would give meaning to my life. How did B.J. Adams know about me and seek me out? She later told me that she remembered me from last year when I attended the Brazelton lectures. Once again I had been rescued, this time by a specific person but no matter, I was no longer that miserable, unhappy and dissociated old woman of the morning. If romance had been in my life, it had been with my profession, and that had never let me down.

The Adages and Me

The purpose of writing my autobiography was to see if this would reveal how I came to be me, but did it? First, before I answered that question, I had to decide who I was and that meant a self-analysis which was not an easy task. Now, maybe Mark Twain's concepts of the truth would show! Could I be really truthful about myself? I asked. Could I really view myself realistically? Well, I had to try, but how should I start? I thought that I must look at the end result and start with the here and now. I was in those golden years, a polite way of saying, I think, that I was an old woman. Yes, it was true if you counted the years that I had been on this planet, but I had no physical or mental deficits and the 'rheumatism' that I suffered from last year had left me, and I could do most things that I needed to do. Was this the result of following that old adage, 'Early to bed and early to rise, makes a man or woman healthy, wealthy and wise,' I wondered. Certainly the 'healthy' part applied to me.

There was that other old adage, 'Moderation in all things'. Was it because I still followed this advice that I still enjoyed the quality of life that I had been used to all my life? I still enjoyed the daily challenges that I was presented with on arising each new day, and I was able to solve most of them. If I couldn't, I knew the right resources to turn to. Day-to-day living was relatively peaceful and I now had time to 'stand and stare' and this assured me that 'my life was not full of care'. I still enjoyed my social activities, having old friends for dinner and making weekend visits, music, drama, art, reading for relaxation and to pass the time of day, good movies and the theatre. Most of all, I still enjoyed nature in all its aspects, glorious and not so glorious, the seasons as they came and went, the dawn and dusk with their sunrises and sunsets, the sleepings and awakenings, the growing and blossoming of the plants, the migration of the birds. I still loved the old world and its human inhabitants.

There were some things that I could not tolerate in my fellow humans and I had to look at these in this examination, for they were the darker side of my personality and actual being. Stupidity headed the list for it was always accompanied by degradation of the self and others. Fools step in where angels fear to tread, I often thought. I was saddened by its constant promotion and its increasing acceptance. I also hated hypocrisy. I could not tolerate anything that was sham or faux.

As Dad used to say, 'I call a spade a spade', and I have tried to follow his dictum. If I was dissatisfied with any situation involving myself and others I tried to evaluate it from both points of view and discuss the problem rationally and without rancour. Of course, I was not always right, but the resolution usually included ongoing positiveness with the other and no hard feelings left over. However, I would not allow myself to be devalued or degraded. To succumb to that only convinced the other person that he was right and had power over the other one.

I hated conflict just as much as I hated hypocrisy and, for a long time, I followed Mother's dictum of 'Peace at any price'. Then I became willing to agree that there were some situations that called for this. It was only as one matured and developed good judgement that one could decide when to stand up or when to cave in. As Dad also said again, 'One must stand up for one's convictions'. Why have them if one doesn't? This did not have to be an adversarial situation. We did not necessarily have to accept the bad with the good. Rather, we should try to remove the bad and replace it with not only good, but that which was right to ensure its continuity. For was this not what life was all about, a continuing process that changed as change was needed? I thought. The other intolerable aspects of life for me were all those 'dis' words; disobedience, dishonesty, disloyalty, disharmony, to name just a few.

Well, that was the darker side of me and it seemed clear now that it developed from my early life within my unique family. Dad set the tone by living up to all those adages he recited to us, as well as practising his own beliefs. Mother supported him in every way. Their goal was to develop a decent, law-abiding citizen, able to fit in with the demands of society. Yes, that was me. So those old adages worked, but what of the lighter, and brighter side of me?

I was pleasant, friendly and outgoing, reminding me of that old adage of Mother's, 'Smile and the world smiles with you, weep and you weep alone'. As I wrote this, I was reminded of my colleagues at Dudley Road Hospital who called me, 'The girl with the Golden Smile'. Was that the result of that old adage? I was loyal to my friends and associates and I tried to be available to them in their hours of need, as well as at times of fun and pleasure. 'If I'm your friend, I'm your friend,' was my motto, and my friendships of more than half a lifetime seemed to confirm that this had paid off. I was honest and open and I tried to be receptive to new ideas, new methods and new thinking, but I was not easily convinced. Proof had to be available, so that I could evaluate both sides of the coin. This did not allow for spontaneity or impulsiveness. Caution was the name of my game! As I wrote this, that old adage of Mother's rang in my ears, 'Look before you leap'. In my adult life I have benefited from these attributes of good planning, good organising and good management, especially in my professional life, again the result of those old adages that are still ringing in my ears, 'A place for everything and everything in its place'. When I finally convinced my children of this, we noticed how seldom we had to look and search for our daily necessities. I cannot conclude without lauding another of those wise old sayings, 'Give credit where credit is due'. That has earned me many friends and good relationships both at work and play.

Well! I have blown my own trumpet! I wonder how wrong I am. As I read my autobiography again, it seems clear that my personality developed in my early years and as a result of my family life. For my parents lived what they preached and even my extended family members lived and preached the same ideas and values. There was no conflict or confusion for Sis and me. One other notion that they all reinforced was education. Both Mother's family and Dad's conveyed to us that this was the way to go but, most of all, they always portrayed the concept of education positively, through books, games, travel and historical events. No matter what, fun was part of learning and this set us on our paths. As each phase ended, it set the scene and the tone for the next.

Perhaps for me, at least, Mother's refrain of, 'Be independent' was the most vital force driving me on. Her notion, developed from her own experience, gave me great satisfaction and pride as I made it one of my own goals throughout my life. One needs social relationships and friends with loyalty, commitment, respect and common interests, too, and I was lucky, for I had such relationships with both men and women. I must agree that friends were the chocolate chips in the cookie of life for out of such relationships one finds one's own true self and, from one's true self, one finds peace and contentment within one's self.

So, how did I come to be me? The credit must go first of all to my parents and my extended family for sharing their beliefs through the living of them. Those old adages kept coming back and reminding me of the basic rules that we lived by. Others supported my parents and I have to give credit to my teachers too for they reinforced within the classroom all that I was experiencing at home. I cannot forget the graduation speaker urging us 'to go down in the surging foam of the river rather than wallow in the murky waters of the delta'. That helped me in times of change and challenge and promoted me to look for and cope with the latter at times when no solution seemed possible. What of that unknown and unseen force that always came to my rescue at times of transition and change? What was it? – Kismet, Fate, God? I personally believe that it was faith, faith in one's self, faith that one could do it, despite the anxiety, the worry and the fears brought on by the unknown, faith that one could solve whatever needed to be solved and could solve it with a smile. If this was the challenge of life, then I had made it, and made it with pleasure and happiness.

As Leo Buscaglia said in his book, *Papa, My Father*:

> I had much to thank my parents for. They showed me that life was an exciting adventure and challenged me to take full advantage of all that it had to offer. They hooked me on learning and taught me my responsibility for leaving the world a better place for my having been in it. The facts of life they modelled for me were simple. They lived by a positive code, the rules of which were uncomplicated and accessible to anyone wanting to live a good life.

Yes, it had been a good life and now, in the twilight years, let it continue as it will. Thank you Mother and Dad for all your devotion and care, but, most of all, for teaching me those old adages that kept me on my straight and narrow path of life.

Requiem to Oliver

Farewell little fellow who over the years has been my best friend –
   a delight
It has pained me so much to see your fears and be unable to help
   with your plight.

We have spent fifteen years together, good years every one
You were always there when I needed a friend for love, comfort
   and to help me along.
How did you find me my little stray? Was it ordained from above?
No matter the reason, the purpose or chance, you brought me
   glad tidings and love.

Even Pledge, Esther's dog and your half sister, took you into her
   world with acceptance.
She patiently mothered and cared for you and made you a man of
   substance
For you were honest, loyal, tolerant and true and cared greatly for
   your mistress,
You stayed by her side with obvious pride at good times and bad
   times and in crises.

At those times of crisis, you always were there enquiringly seeking
   the reason
With your wonderful eyes so expressive and wise encouraging a
   rational solution.
I really believe that you understood the little refrain and ditty
Oliver, Polliver, what shall we do, that I chanted when in a tizzy.

By jumping down from your cosy couch and coming physically close,
The warmth you conveyed to a saddened old maid restored her lost feelings of hope.
And what did you feel over all these years of happiness sorrow and pain,
Did you sense our acceptance and trust and love? I think so, so our lives were not in vain.

Now you have left me my life is bereft, each day is depressing and blue,
No one could replace you to comfort my heart and help with life's challenges too.
So farewell my old friend, so faithful and true, rest in peace now your journey is over,
We will meet one another again one fine day, and then we'll be back in clover.